Research in Health and Social Care

Research in Health and Social Care equips students and early-career practitioners with the crucial knowledge, skills and understanding required to conduct sound research. Accessibly written, it is structured to allow professionals and students to engage in the theoretical development of their practice in ethical and reflective research.

Each chapter is co-written with students, featuring vignettes from health and social care students that highlight their personal journeys with research engagement. Content includes:

- exploring the everyday nature of research, processes, procedures and analysis;
- demystifying key terminology;
- an introduction to research and its importance in practice;
- creative and traditional tools of research;
- analysing data and how to disseminate data;
- approaches to research;
- embedding research into practice.

Discussions around key theoretical ideas are explored throughout, as well as opportunities for deep reflection.

This essential book is perfect for all social work and health and social care students, as well as early-career practitioners, aiming to deepen their knowledge and skills in conducting robust, ethical and relevant developmental research.

Simon Williams is Head of Discipline for Public Health and Social Care at the University of Derby. Simon is a professional Youth Worker and has extensive experience in working with faith groups, asylum seekers, refugees and economic migrants, particularly the Roma Community. Simon leads a variety of research-based projects, especially around professional practice development, and has a keen passion for practice-based research that is co-produced.

Rachel Searcey is a Lecturer in the Discipline of Public Health and Social Care at the University of Derby. She holds a PhD in Social Science from Loughborough University, where her doctoral research focused on the voice of street-based sex workers' histories of child sexual exploitation, exploring the transitional support from childhood to adulthood. With over 20 years of experience in both the charitable and statutory sectors, and as a qualified youth worker, Rachel has worked extensively with street-based sex workers, young people, families and communities. She remains committed to improving public health and social care outcomes through her teaching practice and research.

Research in Health and Social Care

Edited by
Simon Williams and Rachel Searcey

Routledge
Taylor & Francis Group

LONDON AND NEW YORK

Designed cover image: AdobeStock

First published 2026
by Routledge
4 Park Square, Milton Park, Abingdon, Oxon OX14 4RN

and by Routledge
605 Third Avenue, New York, NY 10158

Routledge is an imprint of the Taylor & Francis Group, an informa business

British Library Cataloguing-in-Publication Data
A catalogue record for this book is available from the British Library

ISBN: 978-1-041-05679-9 (hbk)
ISBN: 978-1-916-92530-4 (pbk)
ISBN: 978-1-041-05678-2 (ebk)

DOI: 10.4324/9781041056782

Typeset in Sabon
by codeMantra

Contents

CONTENTS

Contributors

Michael Balkow is a Social Work Lecturer at the University of Derby, teaching on the MA and BA social work degrees. He is a registered social worker with seven years' experience working across child protection, public and private law family proceedings, children with disabilities and children's mental health.

Dr Paula Beesley is a Senior Lecturer in Social Work at Leeds Beckett University. Her research interests focus primarily on pedagogical exploration of students' experiences of social work education. Her reflective qualitative research often uses narrative inquiry to explore students' experiences to inform practice.

Julie Bernstein is a Senior Occupational Therapy Lecturer at the University of Derby. She qualified as an Occupational Therapist in 2000 and completed a National Institute for Health Research funded MA in Research Methods in 2011 at the University of Nottingham. She has been teaching about research to health and social care students since 2013.

Dr Chloe Blackwell is a research associate at the Centre for Research in Social Policy, Loughborough University. Her work explores the needs and financial experiences of different household types. She conducts regular focus groups and interviews with adults and children in many different circumstances that impact household income and expenditure requirements.

Esme Blood, a graduate of the University of Derby's Dance & Choreography Master's programme, works with Adaire to Dance, Liminal Dance Collective and StandBack DanceCo. She delivers movement sessions across Derby, promoting dance for mental and physical well-being, combining technical expertise with a passion for creativity and community engagement.

Emily Currell is a graduate of the University of Derby and obtained a first degree in Youth and Community Work, with a Pathway in SEND. She started her career in faith-based practice and has worked between education, youth clubs and informal youth work settings. Her key interests are working alongside SEND individuals and she wants to focus on improving education for them to better cater for their needs within a neurotypical environment.

Dr Lesley Deacon is Associate Professor of Practice Research at the University of Sunderland. She is also an NIHR ARC NENC Social Care Research Fellow, Social Care Speciality Co-lead for the RRDN and a registered social worker. Her areas of interest are practice research, neurodiversity and safeguarding.

Charlotte Domanski trained with the Frontline social work programme, qualifying in 2022 and gaining a Masters in 2023 with the dissertation topic of engaging extended family networks. She has worked in assessment and long-term support teams within Children's Social Care at an inner London borough.

Dr Melanie Durowse is a Social Work Lecturer at University of Dundee. Previously she has worked in statutory child care, foster care and more recently in adult social work. Her research interests are adult protection, financial harm, how judgements and decisions are made in social work.

Jessica Eve Jackson is an Associate Professor in the Centre of Children and Young People's Health at the University of Nottingham. She has over 20 years of nursing experience in various health and social care settings. Her research fosters community collaboration and explores complexities around key public health priorities.

Dr Dolapo Fakuade (Dolas) is a 'pracademic' with over a decade teaching, training and working experience in academic institutions and public sector organisations in the UK, USA, New Zealand, Australia, Singapore, Turkey and United Arab Emirates. She leads the Intelligence, Security and Disaster Management MSc at the University of Derby.

Dr Julius Gane is a wellbeing worker with Shared Lives, Leeds City Council undertaking a social work apprenticeship at Leeds Beckett University. Whilst he holds a PhD in Bioenergy, he now aims to build on his academic experience in developing a relevant career path within social work practice.

Var Gibson came to University of Dundee from Ukraine when her studies were interrupted by the war. She successfully completed her MSc and is now working as a social worker in Angus Council. Var has a strong interest in social justice and became interested in research through working with people diagnosed with dementia.

Dr Tessa Godfrey is a registered social worker and a Lecturer at the University of Greenwich. Her doctoral research explored students' experiences of completing action research. She has also contributed to research relating to systemic supervision.

Jenni Guthrie is a registered social worker, Principal Curriculum Lead at Frontline and is completing a professional doctorate in social work with Tavistock and Portman NHS Trust. She is a published author and a peer reviewer for *Practice* and the *British Journal of Social Work*.

Antonette Hall is a dedicated Health Inequalities Outreach Practitioner at Family Support Link, providing essential support to families affected by their loved one's substance misuse. She earned a first-class bachelor's degree in Applied Social Care and Education Studies and a distinction for her Masters in Education Studies from the University of Northampton. Her research focuses on societal and educational inequalities with a strong advocacy for race, equality and diversity. Antonette received the 2022 Innovations in Research Award for Best Academic Research.

Carrie Harrop is a PhD researcher in social policy at Loughborough University. Her study explores the financial needs and transitions of care leavers. She has more than ten years of experience working with care leavers and young people in care.

Dr Sarah Henderson is a Principal Lecturer, and Applied Social Sciences Course Leader, in the School of Law and Social Sciences at the Robert Gordon University, Aberdeen. Sarah has taught research methods and quantitative analysis techniques to undergraduate and postgraduate students from various health and social care backgrounds.

Dean Howard is a care leaver and recent graduate of Youth Work and Community Development in the Youth Justice Pathway. His career began as a care leaver with a personal experience of youth work, which led into a professional career. His professional interests are based in safeguarding, prevent and holistic interventions and counselling through games and development.

Jay Jones is a final year BSc Occupational Therapy student at the University of Derby, with lived experience as a child in care and within specialist education. As an OT student, he has developed research interests in Neurological Rehabilitation, Hand Therapy & Interoception differences within individuals with autism.

Dr Rhiannon Jones (FRSA) is Associate Professor (Civic Practice) and Head of Civic and Communities, University of Derby, and a thought leader in creative placemaking. She founded Designing Dialogue CIC, that runs S.H.E.D, a model of best practice for British Council, Council for Higher Education in Art and Design, National Centre for Academic and Cultural Exchange. She leads CivicLAB at the University of Derby and Chairs Cumulus Global Association Contemporary Art Group.

Tess King is an experienced independent social work practitioner and manager with 20 years of safeguarding, specialising in Harmful Sexual Behaviour (HSB). She provides assessments, interventions, training and consultations nationally. Her focus is on HSB, child sexual abuse and supporting professionals with tailored training, policies and service development.

Mel Lindley is Head of School for Allied Health and Social Care at the University of Derby. Mel's research spans the development and validation of self-assessment questionnaires in clinical practice and pedagogic research, exploring the impact and experiences of different learning technologies (simulation, virtual reality), through mixed methods approaches.

Alice Marshall (Vale), founder of Adaire to Dance, is a distinguished artist, educator and Routledge-published author. As SFHEA and Programme Leader for BA and MA Dance programmes, she champions innovation in performing arts. Her global influence spans choreography, education and research, supported by Arts Council-funded touring performances.

Jessica Millington is a Clinical Lead Occupational Therapist with over ten years' experience, specialising in Adult Community Mental Health. She has worked extensively in facilitating and supporting student placements in this field. She has completed an MSc in Advanced Occupational Therapy at the University of Derby.

Professor Matt Padley is Co-Director of the Centre for Research in Social Policy, where he has pioneered work on retirement living standards. He leads research on living standards in London and works across the established Minimum Income Standard programme. His research focuses on public conceptions of living standards, and how these can inform policy.

Amy Payne is a newly qualified social worker, working with people with neurodiverse conditions. Amy's background is working in domiciliary care, and she is passionate about involving families in conversations with professionals. Amy completed her dissertation around the support families receive with a dementia diagnosis.

Lorne Power is a doctoral research fellow based at the University of Sussex, currently researching social care with trans and/or gender non-conforming people with learning difficulties. Their professional experience includes social work, advocacy and commissioning and they are particularly interested in neurodiversity, queer social work and participatory research. Doctoral Local Authority Fellow, NIHR303070 is funded by the NIHR. The views expressed in this publication are those of the author(s) and not necessarily those of the NIHR, NHS or the UK Department of Health and Social Care

Alessia Renganeschi is a final-year MSc Occupational Therapy student at the University of Derby, with a previous background in special education and the Montessori method. As an OT student, she has developed research interests in perinatal and infant mental health and co-occupation, early childhood occupation and development, and Montessori-based therapeutic practices.

Dr Rachel Searcey is a Lecturer in the Discipline of Public Health and Social Care at the University of Derby. She holds a PhD in Social Science from Loughborough University, where her doctoral research focused on the voice of street-based sex workers' histories of child sexual exploitation, exploring the transitional support from childhood to adulthood. With over 20 years of experience in both the charitable and statutory sectors, and as a qualified youth worker, Rachel has worked extensively with street-based sex workers, young people, families and communities. She remains committed to improving public health and social care outcomes through her teaching practice and research.

Agnella Serafin combines expertise in finance, technology and psychology. Currently working in the asset management sector, she holds an MSc in Applied Psychology and two economics degrees. As a former entrepreneur, she developed VR-driven mental well-being solutions, advancing innovation and fostering interdisciplinary connections throughout her professional journey.

Mandy Simpson is a social worker who has a keen interest in supporting older adults. Her interest in research began during her time at the University of Derby where she was involved in conducting and presenting primary research on women's biopsychosocial experiences during perimenopause and menopause. Mandy is delighted to contribute her thoughts and reflection from a student perspective within this book.

Leanne Skanta-Reading is a qualified Nurse and Program Leader for Nursing and Health Care Practice at the University of Derby. Leanne's interests lie in health promotion, with a focus on sexual health care and reproductive services. Leanne's Masters degree in health and social care focused on the impact and consequences of sexual violence on survivors. Transitioning from the NHS to academia has allowed Leanne to inspire and educate the next generation of healthcare professionals while sharing a passion for patient care.

Hazel Spence holds an MSc from the University of Bradford. Her professional experience as an advanced practitioner in radiology at Nottingham University hospitals inspired her to undertake a Masters degree focusing on evaluating the efficacy of computed tomography pulmonary angiograms as a diagnostic tool for detecting pulmonary embolisms in pregnant patients.

Robin Sturman-Coombs is a registered and experienced social worker, educator, trainer, researcher and leader with expertise in safeguarding, mental health and social care. Prior to academia, he spent time working in Child Protection and Safeguarding, managing complex Child Protection Cases from Referral through to Initial Court Hearing. His passion for social work has led to an emerging interest in how HEIs prepare students to practice intuitive reasoning in social work practice, and he has a deep interest in attachment, bonding and relationships. Robin teaches from foundation to Masters level study and is in the final stages of his own doctoral studies. He is an independent trainer with a specialism in fostering and adoption.

Chantelle Taylor is a PhD candidate in the Department of Sociology and Social Policy at Loughborough University. She is a qualitative researcher using autoethnography and reflexive thematic analysis to explore hidden mothering and the role of online peer support in navigating societal expectations of motherhood.

Ola Tony-Obot is an Equity, Diversity and Inclusion Lead at Together for Children, Sunderland; a senior social work practitioner and researcher; practice educator; public speaker and cultural competence trainer. Her research explores areas in social care and cultural competence. She has knowledge in conducting and analysing research of varied methods.

Helen Turrell is a third-year social work student at the University of Derby. Helen has spent the last decade raising her four children and became passionate about pursuing a career in social work following her experience of working in children's homes and in hospitals.

Cynthia Tuuli is a Social Work Lecturer at the University of Derby. Her research interests are around minority students' experiences in higher education and the attainment gap, and in understanding the lived experiences of peri- and menopausal women. Cynthia also has social work experience in working with vulnerable adults.

Kay Wall is a Senior Lecturer at the University of Worcester. She also holds the role of IMPACT facilitator, the university's experts by experience group. She is passionate about listening to the voices of people with lived experience to improve social work practice and research.

Rachel Watts is a social worker in an Inner London Child Protection service. She completed a Masters in Relationship Based Social Work practice, researching ways to better advocate for and reflect the voices of children with limited speech development, considering barriers to inclusion and the benefits of multi-disciplinary working.

Thomas Wheatley has recently graduated from the University of Derby with a degree in Youth Work and Community Development. Since graduating, Thomas has secured a job within the pastoral team of a high achieving secondary school, working with the safeguarding and senior leadership teams to support students academically and personally.

Simon Williams is Head of Discipline for Public Health and Social Care at the University of Derby. Simon is a professional Youth Worker and has extensive experience in working with faith groups, asylum seekers, refugees and economic migrants, particularly the Roma Community. Simon leads a variety of research-based projects, especially around professional practice development, and has a keen passion for practice-based research that is co-produced.

Figures

Tables

Introduction

Simon Williams and Rachel Searcey

Health and social care is a diverse field that involves a variety of practitioners, volunteers and academics from a range of professions that seek to support individuals, groups and communities to 'live their best life'. The extent of this professional practice across the field provides an array of experience, understanding and application through interprofessional and multiagency working. However, this can also present challenges such as value clashes, priorities and funding outcomes, which can impact on effective health and social care research.

This edited collection recognises that research can often be contested and a difficult topic to comprehend, develop and be critical about; notwithstanding implementing the changes in everyday practice. Many practitioners have different personal priorities and interests that hone their research focus. For some, their professional and personal values impact their sense of direction. Additionally, the pull of managerialism, funding and outcomes equally drives the research agenda as does the impact of policy, government agendas, public health crisis and more. All of this means that research is pulled in many directions and can be seen as aloof and not related to practice. This can often lead many to be critical of the research processes.

As students studying research, the concept can often seem like a mammoth beast that is impossible to understand, wrestle with and deliver. No matter what stage of your higher education journey you are in, research (which seems to have its own language) can often seem intimidating and exclusive. There can be a sense of academic snobbery that can impact research delivery and practice, which also means that many practitioners avoid research. Many practitioners who have studied at higher education will have engaged in some form of research within their practice. Yet the embedding and application of research in practice is affected by the culture and attitude of other researchers and practitioners who have individual histories of engaging in research (sometimes negative). However, what is known is that research is impactful. Research ultimately impacts on all areas of health and social care practice, from government and policy choices to the everyday connection between practitioners and service users, the

DOI: 10.4324/9781041056782-1

types of medication and responses to certain issues to the public's opinion of social care and health issues.

Therefore, this edited collection has been designed and organised to support student and practitioner researchers to help plan, action and evaluate effective research processes. For this to be of value to students, the editors agreed that certain aspects were needed:

- Student voice and co-creation of chapters
- Reflective questioning
- Diverse field representation

Each chapter has been co-created with at least one higher education student, who is a currently active student or within one year of graduating (at the time of writing). The students have been involved in the whole chapter writing process so that their voice is included throughout each chapter. Some authors are undergraduates, some master level and others doctoral level. There is also a student voice section in each chapter, where the student takes more of a 'talking to the reader' approach, which enables students to explore their experiences and responses to the aspects discussed in the chapter. When the editors explored this as a key aspect of the book, students fed back that they did not always want to be identified directly as students, so we have taken this approach, although some students were happy to be identified as such in the student voice section. This co-creation approach has enriched the writing process, making sure that each chapter is written in an appropriate way to support understanding, be of use to students for their own academic writing and of use for practitioner-researchers to enact in practice.

Reflective questions have been added in each chapter. These are designed to help the reader reflect and respond to the content. We hope the readers of this edited collection will be active in testing the ideas and theories (and building on them) in their own practice and we hope the questions will enable you to do this. We wanted a book that was based on theory and supported readers to see theory in action. Specifically, we want our readers to see how theory can be understood, applied and critiqued to support practice, and by actioning these theories this would create more research and development of newer theories.

With health and social care being such a broad field of practice, we wanted to make sure we had a wide range of authors across the health and social care field to represent a wide variety of experiences and application of theory. As such we have authors involved in a range of practices from social work to nursing, public health to youth work. We think this adds to the richness of the book. We have sought to keep a universal approach around language throughout, this has meant using some terms that might create some debate but are often wider understood. For example, we use the term 'service user' throughout as this is a universally understood term, but we do also recognise that this term can be problematic.

The book's design has been set out to take the reader through the research journey; we have split the book into three parts:

- Preparing the ground for research
- Designing your research project
- Evaluating your research and understanding the wider implications

Chapter 1 sets out the scene for the book, recognising the impact of power on research practice. The chapter sets out an exploration of power in academic research, and how it can be seen as something aloof to practitioners. The chapter debates the power of individuals involved in research and recognising the power of the student researcher, but also the power of others that can impact a student researcher; it uses theory to help support the reader to reflect on their own power. The chapter supports thinking that leads to effective reflective practice around power, including ideologies that powerfully affect research practice such as anti-intellectualism but also the role of the student researcher as challenging power.

Chapter 2 examines historical research practice and the significant impact this has had on current practice and research. It defines what research is and usefully highlights some pioneers in research practice and how this practice has been critiqued and developed to make sure participants are fully respected. The chapter debates the role of anti-oppressive practice in research and challenges the reader to be critical in their approach to sources to develop new ways of working. The chapter highlights practices researchers can be involved in to develop their research practice such as journal clubs and peer review.

Chapter 3 continues the discussion towards evidence-based research to explore the connection of research on society. It debates the potential clashes between research and practice and questions the use of 'common sense', highlighting the need for practice to be informed by research. The chapter seeks to connect research practice with development of service and the role of scrutiny to create change. The chapter debates the impact of research on policy making and how much wider, national decisions are framed around evidence-based practice. The chapter encourages the reader to identify, integrate and interrogate evidence to support practice that is of high quality and able to respond to the diverse needs of its service users.

Chapter 4 directs the reader to explore the role of ethics, underpinned by the previous three chapters' discussions. The chapter debates moral history and governance as a contested and complex field, so sets out the ethical journey for the researcher journey. The chapter supports reflective practice within research, recognising the potential conflicts within practices of researchers, practitioners and service users. The chapter helpfully sets out how to work with and respond to ethics committees to maintain inclusive practice balanced with power dynamics. The chapter also discusses consent and some of the barriers to this. The chapter will support the reader to make use of 'self' to recognise ethical practice, to build confidence as a researcher and build trust with participants in your research.

Chapter 5 focuses on how the researcher's identity shapes the relationship with research, participants, readers and the ivory tower. This chapter specifically highlights how the researcher's lived experience can challenge the internal and external biases and promote positive collaboration to foster inclusive outcomes. One key theme in this chapter is reflexivity; this brings close attention to researcher participation and inclusion of their own personal experiences and journeys for the enhancement of knowledge and research.

Chapter 6 presents a discussion on reflexive and flexible research across the field of health and social care. The authors consider how reflection can enhance ethical research and aids a flexible approach to research when working with vulnerable people within health and social care research. This chapter provides a series of helpful tools to support reflection through the research journey through the use of a reflective research diary and how to effectively engage with research supervisors. The chapter concludes by considering the importance of flexible research within the research process, particularly reflecting on the needs of people with lived experience who participate in research projects.

Chapter 7 sets a discussion around the involvement of participants who may be described as vulnerable. The chapter helps the reader recognise participants as an important part of the research journey and advises on how to work with potential issues when working with those described as vulnerable. The chapter recognises research as part of the social context, and how the experience of participants adds value to the research planning, implementation and analysis of research. The chapter discusses mental capacity of participants and how to include a range of diverse participants, but recognises the challenges that working creatively can raise. The chapter champions coproduction at all stages of the research journey in a way that is not tokenistic.

Chapter 8 debates the benefits of involving people with lived experiences in research. It critically argues how organisational and institutional barriers affect how people with lived experiences view and experience research if not actively involved in the research processes. The authors encourage the reader to interrogate the reasons for adopting a more traditional approach to research when excluding people with lived experiences. They approach this important aspect by highlighting the power dynamics that exist between the researcher and those who are 'researched'. Across this chapter, there is a clear and valid argument for researchers to adopt a more active approach to research through collaboration by involving people with lived experiences. The chapter is both insightful and informative, giving a balanced view for a collaborative approach to research.

Chapter 9 examines the role of secondary data and how it can inform and develop practice. The chapter debates the challenges and benefits of secondary research and offers tools to consider in a research journey. The chapter sets out the differences between primary and secondary research and encourages the reader to see the lived experiences through secondary research. The chapter demonstrates how a qualitative secondary research study can be approached, providing a variety of tools and resources to support the researcher to start their journey into secondary research. The chapter concludes that secondary research has a critical role in research practice, providing a systematic method for data collection and analysis.

Chapter 10 starts by providing an overview of research philosophies and paradigms to help the reader understand the theoretical underpinnings that shape and form the design of any research project. The methodologies of qualitative, mixed-methods and quantitative approaches are then introduced to the reader. The chapter concludes with a range of qualitative research methods with practical advice and considerations of how to apply these in practice. This chapter is particularly helpful for students who are unsure of how theory connects directly to the methods of data collection.

Chapter 11 debates the use of creative methods in gathering data. The chapter supports the use of creative methods and explores some of the limitations involved in both creative and more traditional methods. The chapter usefully discusses the political and social context that impacts on research methods, and how tools can be a powerful limiting factor, as well as a powerful enhancer, to individual voices. The chapter highlights the connection of the impact of austerity and the environment on how researchers approach gathering data. The chapter discusses the authors' use of Q sort as a creative method to support their research working with people with dementia, which highlights some of the critical development the authors have gone through in their own research journey.

Chapter 12 provides essential tips and guidance on creative placemaking through student led curriculum design. Taking the reader on a journey from ideation to the installation of creative practices within a clinical research context, to developing new ecosystems for knowledge transfer with the public. The chapter provides tips on how to integrate scientific data into the delivery of artistic and design led outputs, leading to influencing policy through creative placemaking, and the role of sci-art practice as a tool for social mobility and improved healthcare provisions and awareness. The benefits and challenges of co-designing with stakeholders in the public realm with Designing Dialogue CIC, that delivers the project S.H.E.D, is explored, and how it embedded clinical research seamlessly into artistic installation.

Chapter 13 focuses on the practical, theoretical and ethical issues that are key to the processes of data analysis and research dissemination. Centred around first-person action research as a methodology, the chapter considers forms of analysis focusing specifically on reflexive thematic analysis. It then explores how dissemination needs to be continually considered throughout the entire research process. The authors consider how values of social justice can be incorporated into research, through collaborative and creative approaches to data analysis and dissemination. The authors have thoughtful and creative approaches to analysis and dissemination not only to benefit the researcher, but also research participants and the communities in which they live.

Chapter 14 ends the collection looking at the current picture of health and social care practice. It highlights the impact of systems in responding to health and social care issues, calling for students and practitioners to be active in research to highlight and respond to issues. The chapter debates how the political, economic and social climate impact the work and research field of health and social care, highlighting the social determinates of health and how these are interconnected and yet framed within political discourse. The chapter calls for responses to be made to change the social inequalities that are experienced and seek to provide services which widen participation.

It is the editors' hopes that this edited collection is useful to both the student and practitioner equally in developing their confidence to engage in research, providing the evidence that creates significant and real change in organisational practice, policy making and government decisions to support individuals and communities to live their best life.

PART I

Preparing the ground for research

Power in research

Simon Williams, Dean Howard, Emily Currell and Thomas Wheatley

Introduction

'But sir, why do I need to learn the quadratic formula? How is this going to help me?' A variation on this conversation is repeated in classrooms worldwide, where young people may feel forced to learn things because adults have told them to. From our days in education, we learn about power and who holds it. For some students in health and social care studies the idea of 'power' can be quite removed from their current thinking and experiences. Health and social care practice is embedded in anti-oppressive practice, recognising and responding to abuses of power, and so should any related research practices. However, for some, our personal, cultural, and structural experiences can lead us to become 'blind' to certain issues and leave some aspects of power imbalance unchallenged. Students, practitioners, and academics alike must wrestle with the concept of power when looking at research (Gravlee, 2020; Sunderland et al, 2022).

This chapter provides an overview of 'power', looking at the various forms that can affect positive research practice, through examining how theory affects practice. It focuses on critically examining the 'ivory tower', positionality, and anti-intellectualism to see how these concepts impact research.

Chapter concepts
This chapter addresses these three concepts across four areas:

- Academic research power;
- Individual research power;
- Ideological research power;
- The effect of power on research practice.

Power

When discussing power, we are talking about all aspects of practice that can be perceived as an imbalance of power. For instance, practitioners' body language,

DOI: 10.4324/9781041056782-3

communication methods, or the cultural attitudes of practitioners. It can also be structural and seen in policy (Beattie, 2003; Cain et al, 2018).

Reflective question

As you read this chapter, we suggest you reflect on the following. How can you recognise your situation and power and how does it affect you and your practice?

Academic research

Academics can be seen as distant, removed from the realities of practice; this is the concept of the 'ivory tower' (Mulholland, 2015; Rawlins, 2019), which suggests that academics in their isolated universities do not know the 'real' world of practice. As such, practitioners sometimes perceive a gulf between the 'ivory tower' of academic theory and the 'trenches' of health and social care practice (Tolsgaard et al, 2020). Yet, there is some benefit to being removed from practice when undertaking research. For academics and policymakers, this separation from practice ensures they refrain from 'fitting' theories and research to the current political context (Nye, 2008; Lepgold and Nincic, 2001). Academics (including university students) can be perceived to be in a privileged position, viewed as possessing the most current knowledge and theory for best practice.

Nye (cited in Byman and Kroenig, 2016, p 289) commented that 'the walls surrounding the ivory tower never seemed so high'. A similar situation is represented within the UK Government Department of Health and Social Care. Current Secretary of State Steve Barclay has 'no known experience in health or social care, having trained as a solicitor and worked in finance before becoming an MP' and is supported by a permanent (and second permanent) secretary, who has no health and social care experience. Although the role of a government minister differs from the role of an academic, there is some common ground in the power imbalances on display. Therefore, a bridge needs to be made across this sizeable gap between practice, policy, and academia (Nursing Notes, 2022).

Jentleson and Ratner (2011) suggest that 'policy-relevant scholarship' is the best option for narrowing the divide between practice and academia. Policy-relevant scholarship aims to make research explicit in its intention to respond to gaps in practice and create responses. This could potentially create a more balanced power dynamic, allowing practitioners and policymakers to identify a need for theoretical support and allowing academics to provide it directly. Additionally, the involvement of service users in research design is key to developing practice and theories that support the beneficiaries of services (Veldmeijer et al, 2023; Barber et al, 2011).

Research should be impacted by all parties who benefit, but this can be time-consuming and potentially risky. Practitioners and service users might struggle with complex research philosophies but will be able to equalise power dynamics to form foundations to build a functional and effective service.

To allow each member to have involvement at any stage of the research project, individuals need to examine their power; a key aspect of this is considering a concept called positionality.

Individual research power

Student Placement assessments can provide research opportunities within a structured, often predetermined, aim. However, what motivates a student's reasons for conducting research can be the student's positionality. Hall (1990) describes positionality as the concept of speaking and writing due to specific events and experiences in your life; these experiences and histories form a positional view of the world. Your position defines your viewpoint and thoughts about people, places, and more. The impact positionality has on a student's research experience may very well build the foundation on which the research is conducted (Holmes, 2020). A student's position may begin to change when qualitative or quantitative data is found that contradicts or reaffirms the student's beliefs and ideas. Students are impacted by their previous experiences and the conflict between their beliefs and research outcomes. We as authors have experienced this change of position. University is commonly a transitional period in a student's life; coming from varying backgrounds and cultures, with different life experiences, can present new challenges, opportunities, and relationships in the university context. All of these culminate in new self-expressions, interests, and identities (Krause and Coates, 2008 in Hoi, 2023).

In a study by Elander et al (2010), it is noted that younger students arriving at university often 'cling' to familiar social structures that they see as relevant and important to them; ie race, faith, or gender (Attinasi, 1989, in Elander et al, 2010, p 7). These may be viewed as fixed aspects. A response to these forms of positionality may be for students to align themselves with new and diverse individuals, groups, and opportunities to challenge their existing positionality. This aspect of mobility, mobilising into new networks and maintaining existing networks, is a valuable journey, although can contain conflict and upset. Students can become resistant to mobility and instead cling to the comfort of peer and environmental familiarity and miss out on wider and sometimes challenging learning. Changing positionality is an ongoing and ever-changing process. Bengtsson et al (2020, p 1) refer to transitions as 'the sense of leaving one social position for another'. Notwithstanding social class or economic background, students often have a variety of university experiences to foster challenge to positionality.

Students are experts in their own lives; this shared expertise can make universities valuable places of learning where power can be shared. The term 'expert by experience' (EBE) is frequently used in practice (CQC, 2023). Being an EBE denotes that the service user's lived experience of events and/or services offers unique insights, thus uniquely shaping their positionality. This offers students coming to university a valuable and unique opportunity to use their positionality and experience to shape their studies and practice, as well as offering insights for their peers. However, Horgan et al (2020, p 555) further state that despite the importance and value of EBE, without qualifications or suitability the EBE student or practitioner faces clear barriers to success. Students who are EBE might have often experienced a lack of power, and this may be exemplified in undertaking research. Despite this, individuals can mobilise their EBE positionality and thrive. Schemas – individual mental frameworks that attach aspects, views, and concepts of the self to new experiences (Pritchard, 2017) – are integral to mobilisation of positionality. For example, the student practitioner may recognise traits within the people they work with which they have seen or experienced, and so be better placed to support them moving forward. With the correct acknowledgements and

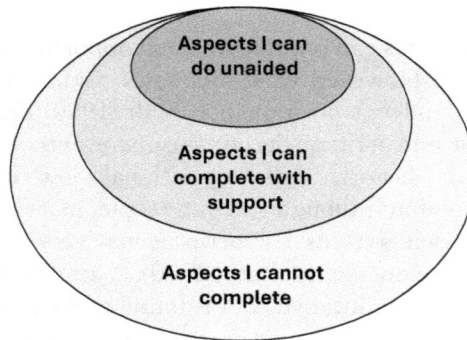

Figure 1.1 Example of Zones of Proximal Development

utilisations of schemas, students can use their positionality, be it coming from a place of EBE or not, to challenge their viewpoints when engaging in research.

Zones of Proximal Development

One tool students can use to reflect on their positionality in research is Vygotsky's Zone of Proximal Development (ZPD) (1978, in Gregson et al, 2015). Vygotsky's ZPD theory (see Figure 1.1) explores the potential to develop and support learning throughout time and place. The medical versus social model (Pilgrim and Rogers, 2005 in Williams and Conroy, 2022) presents varying degrees of conflict for students. For example, when supporting a young client, a student nurse may focus on underlying or present health conditions, whereas a student youth worker may focus on the personal or social events throughout their life. Each student would be correct in their positionality and practice. However, when both reflect on the ZPD model, each student can utilise each other's knowledge and expertise to help grow their positionality and awareness. Furthermore, when both students have reflected on their positionality, and grown their ZPDs, each can create better research findings, providing important outcomes for research.

Without reflective action, diverse positionalities could create a sense of superiority, with some practitioners feeling as though their profession holds more importance in research practice, leading to potential conflict with professionals fighting for importance. Recognising bias, however, is a crucial step in developing unbiased research. Each aspect of health and social care is crucial, and each student and professional needs to remain unbiased and reflective of themselves and others (Hean et al, 2009; Marmor, 2006).

Research practice

Effective research practice is built on the recognition of power, both academic and individual power. Critical discussions are essential in combatting unequal power to develop practice during a research journey. These aspects can be developed in the higher education (HE) environment, through both formal (eg presentations and viva assessments) and informal (eg study groups, coffee breaks, trips) learning journeys. Students are encouraged to wrestle with theory and its application to practice. It is through this wrestling that work is refined and improved, leading to best practice delivery.

Bradford and Cullen (2013) argue that it is important that you recognise yourself as a subject of power and possible coercion. Therefore, research requires effective communication to challenge potential bias and power imbalances. Having a range of communication 'tools' – such as active listening, self-awareness, and sensitivity to the situation – assists in developing relationships (Thompson, 2015) and supporting students in acquiring information in a non-invasive way, for example the use of non-leading questions when acquiring information from participants. Professionals who undertake research within their place of practice may be seen to have an advantage as they already know the participants. Appleby (2014) argues that when there is an existing relationship between researcher and participant this can impact the information that is shared. This allows practitioners to develop a professional bond to enhance communication, although the data can often be more subtle and require deeper examination. Searcey (2022) promotes aiming to avoid tokenistic approaches but developing a genuine sensitive connection suggesting the need for participants to know about us, as we enter their lives with probing questions and interest. Development of effective relationships can help combat power imbalances.

Recognising that being a professional makes us influential people, who service users may aspire to as role models, it may be easy to subconsciously colonise participants, which Belton (2010) describes as directing the participants to think and act in a specific way, often to meet society's ideas of 'good citizens'. This could lead individuals we work with to adopt positionalities that are transferred from practitioners and not necessarily based on their own experiences. Wood et al (2014) agree that it is important for students to be self-aware, examining their ethics, morals, and values to ensure ideologies are not being directly or indirectly imprinted onto service users. Alldred et al (2018) suggest that professionals must be able to question their own power and political views within their practice to enable them to put the interests of service users first. Gormally and Coburn (2014) agree that researchers should not engage in interactions that promote imbalances of power but should instead use reflection to positively enhance research practice. The process of reflective practice is vast, and many models exist, but all seek to raise self-awareness in practitioners. However, reflection needs time, space, and place to be effective. While this might be accomplished during supervision, students need to make sure sufficient time is allocated (Alldred et al, 2018; de St Croix, 2016). Without reflection on an individual's power, ideologies can create bias; reflective practice and good communication can enable students to develop confidence in challenging oppressive ideologies.

Ideological research power

As a teenager, I would sit for hours memorising all the facts needed for an exam. I would then regurgitate all that information onto an exam paper and as I left the exam room, I also left all that memorised knowledge behind. There was a need to demonstrate my ability and I knew this, but the information had no value to me personally. Many students at university may act similarly. Engaging in research and theory is a requirement to pass their degree, and some students may disengage from the learning and knowledge, instead aiming to just pass. This approach to learning relates to the idea of surface and deep learning (Dolmans et al, 2016; Beattie et al, 2010; Dyer and Hurd, 2016). A surface learner will take what they need to pass a test and then leave

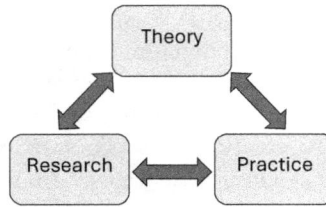

Figure 1.2 Theory to research model

the knowledge behind. An individual involved in deep learning will seek to fully understand the information and apply it to practice, finding a connection. Many aspects affect an individual's ability and attitude to deep learning, including their relationship with the lecturer/teacher, the environment, personal life factors, and more. However, there is the potential in long-term practice for practitioners to develop an attitude (positive or negative) towards education. Some practitioners viewed their education as a step to a higher wage/position. Others consider education pointless as it adds no value: to know how to do the job – you just need to do it. These attitudes are also reflected in the wider media (Peat, 2017; Phillips, 2021; Phillpott, 2022). However, to provide best practice, that is developmental, critical, challenges the status quo, and provides better outcomes, it needs to be married to research and theory (Williams and Conroy, 2022). It should be the case that theory supports practice, which supports research, which challenges theory. This is represented in Figure 1.2.

Anti-intellectualism
For many vocational professions, there can be a sentiment of anti-intellectualism. Anti-intellectualism has been defined as a 'general antagonism directed towards intellectual activities and disdain towards theorists seen as members of an elitist class dwelling in universities ivory towers' (Racine and Vanderberg, 2021).

At its extreme, anti-intellectualism has been used as a political tool to combat critical thinking (Peters, 2018). Eigenberger and Sealander (2001) developed a scale to measure anti-intellectualism in university students, asking participants to rank statements like 'College is a necessary evil', 'value learning for its own sake', and 'some professors are too intellectual'. It is useful for students undertaking university courses to reflect on why they are undertaking their course, as this motivational factor impacts engagement and future practice. Universities and students have a responsibility to support learners to engage in deep thinking about practice to avoid the risk of anti-intellectualism stifling creative practice – ultimately leading to poorer outcomes for service users. The concept of anti-intellectualism can be a powerful factor in practice and the development of staff and practice, leaving concepts of research to academics and seeing research as something aloof, instead of an active and essential part of day-to-day practice.

The concept of research should be a foundational aspect of practice, especially as the student mobilises from university to the workplace (Cohen et al, 2018; Lochmiller and Lester, 2017; Stuart et al, 2016). There is a need for students to be able to challenge anti-intellectualism as they encounter it, whether that is the lecturer, topic, or institution. However, many students might feel oppressed by such attitudes as they are a part of the 'intellectual' system.

Hard-to-reach groups

Other ideologies that hold power in research practice can be concepts such as 'hard-to-reach' groups. Doherty et al (2004) define these as minority groups that are often missed by services and generally do not participate, but different groups of potential participants may also be seen as hard-to-reach because they are not easily accessible by researchers. However, the reason individuals might not participate can be due to traumatic experiences, mistrusting those in any position of power, and not understanding the processes, outcomes, and purpose of research. Searcey (2022) highlights aspects of power by commenting that participants are not passive, but active agents with shifting elements of choice. Often in practice, practitioners are heavily involved with hard-to-reach groups, having professional relationships with individuals and groups that can go beyond an outcome, being significantly invested in people's lives and their journeys (McGinn and Burns, 2023; Moss, 2017; Purcell, 2022).

Research practice

Practitioners within the health and social care field of practice should have developed a vast array of methods to communicate and work alongside those seen as hard to reach, which will be essential for providing effective and engaging research. Unclear communication could lead to groups and individuals mistrusting other professionals and could be potentially harmful as community members disengage from services (Ponterotto and Grieger, 2007; Gyamfi, 2020). For example, in my practice working with the Roma community, there were many organisations, funders, and researchers that wanted to engage with this hard-to-reach group. They often failed to understand the systematic and historical oppression faced by the community; they often failed to understand the impact of being 'strangers' in the country in which they lived; and they often failed to recognise cultural aspects and importance of the family. Therefore, it is important that research is well planned (Chapter 6), ethical (Chapter 7), and has clear outcomes and evaluative processes (Chapter 13). It is also vital that research is flexible and adaptable to meet the needs of participants.

Students are well-placed to challenge oppressive practices and ideologies while on placement and engaged in research. Many agencies that work with students do so because they recognise the value of having a student. However, there can be several expectations of students: that they will have up-to-date knowledge of theory, be critical and challenging of practice, and will develop both themselves and others professionally. This is often the opposite of how students feel. Sometimes students are concerned about being critical and challenging oppressive practices for fear of the impact on their grades (Williams and Conroy, 2022a; Thyberg, 2022). This challenge is, therefore, best explored by students and supervisors making sure they set out expectations and boundaries. Universities should be providing the learning to make sure that students are fully equipped to engage with ideologies while on placement and in practice. However, no matter what, it is vital that students challenge oppressive practice, otherwise they are condoning it.

Student voice

As a student, you will experience both primary and secondary research. It is important in both, whether you are conducting the research or simply reading it, to have an awareness of the power dynamics that are in play. One of the biggest pieces of research-related learning that I will take away from my time at university is that research is taking place all around you. As a student, you are a participant in research for the university as an institution and for your course in terms of teaching mechanisms. You will soon realise that much of the power within this research lies with the researcher. If the question isn't asked, then an answer can't be given. So, if the course lead doesn't ask what you think about the course content, how are you supposed to tell them? This is a key idea to take into practice: as a (potential) researcher, you have the power over the data that you collect. Of course, the participants have the power over their responses, but ultimately their responses are dictated by the questions they are asked. It is the responsibility of the researcher, as I have come to understand, to ensure that participants have the maximum power and influence over the research that is being conducted. This includes the process, results, and the subsequent use of the results. How you achieve this is by having a transparent approach to your research project, by empowering respondents to feel confident enough to give you honest and accurate answers, and by providing them with information that is jargon-free so that they understand the process and what their responses will be used for. Doing as much background work and preparation for your research project beforehand as you can, and being open and honest about your approach, gives you a strong base for your research to flow once it has begun. I have learnt that it is also a good idea to have a reliable mentor with whom you can check in regularly regarding your research project. This must be someone who will keep you accountable and ask you (potentially) difficult questions to ensure that you are staying true to yourself, your morals and values, and the ethics of the project. Allowing yourself to be vulnerable and open with your approach opens up opportunities for your mentor to advise on any potential errors or concerns that they may have, to ensure that your research stays on task and to a suitable timeline. Finally, having written deadlines, with some contingency time should you need it, allows you to stay on task and prevents it from dragging on, which is particularly important when participants are involved, as they will have clear start and end dates that they are required for.

Conclusion

Power is an active 'force' that impacts on practice and research in practice, and as such, students and practitioners need to be critically aware of these dynamics. Nevertheless, by students and practitioners acknowledging the power imbalance across our education systems, this can pave the way for critical challenges of the often taken-for-granted ideologies surrounding research in practice. While the ivory tower has advantages in terms of knowledge exchange, it is argued that rebalancing power in research can be enhanced further with the inclusion of active participation of all parties involved in the research processes. It is here where the argument of positionality is most key. Shifting assumptions from service user participation to service user involvement brings this debate of positionality closer to the core of research – 'with' service as opposed to the research 'on'. To enable this political shift for the rebalance of power, a useful tool to challenge this thinking is reflexive practice. However, the caveat to this is allowing time and space.

There are a range of ideologies that impact our practice, yet we argue that anti-intellectualism is at the core. It is critical for students not only to recognise themselves as a force of power and navigate the political landscape of their institution where power is also held, but to equally recognise the power of service users by actively promoting inclusive practice across all aspects of the research journey. Students need to acknowledge and, in some cases, accept that their journey within research may be impacted by power – from the individual student and external forces. Without time and space for reflection to recognise and respond to positionality and the ideological impacts on research practice, students can end up reinforcing the power imbalance through poor practice, which could potentially cause harm to participants. There should be active engagement from students and universities to consider the power imbalances and take action to respond. There is not always the need to eliminate power imbalance, but to make sure that any use of power reduces risk of harm.

Reflective questions

1. Reflect on your learning and how it has changed your position. In what ways has it affected the way you practice?
2. Identify and discuss an area of bias you have that is a barrier to practice and further learning.
3. What helps you be aware of your own power and what helps you work around this?
4. Do you see yourself as a vital person in the research sector? Explain your answer. What would support you more to feel vital?

References

Alldred, P Cullen, F Edwards, K and Fusco, D (2018) *The SAGE Handbook of Youth Work Practice*. New York: SAGE Publications Limited.

Appleby, MM (2014) *The Nature of Practitioner Research: Critical distance, power and ethics*. Available at: https://repository.derby.ac.uk/download/3662897b689c2f05c8cf6b6cac79ff72 8a452ef c6d093a8f2df8316c264e2e8e/368751/Appleby.pdf (accessed 22 September 2023).

Barber, R Beresford, P Boote, J Cooper, C and Faulkner, A (2011) Evaluating the impact of service user involvement on research: a prospective case study. *International Journal of Consumer Studies*, 35: 609–615.

Beattie, G (2003) *Visible Thought*. London: Routledge.

Beattie, V Collins, B and McInnes, B (2010) Deep and surface learning: a simple or simplistic dichotomy? *Accounting Education*, 6(1): 1–12.

Belton, B (2010) Colonised youth. *Youth and Policy Journal*. Available at: www.youthandpolicy.org/articles/colonised-youth/ (accessed 4 October 2023).

Bengtsson, M Sjöblom, Y and Öberg, P (2020) Transitional patterns when leaving care – Care Leaver's agency in a longitudinal perspective. *Children and Youth Services Review*, 118. Available at: www-sciencedirect-com.ezproxy.derby.ac.uk/science/article/pii/S0190740920311269

Bradford, S and Cullen, F (2013) *Research and Research Methods for Youth Practitioners*. Oxfordshire: Routledge.

Byman, D. and Kroenig, M. (2016) Reaching Beyond the Ivory Tower: A how to Manual. Security Studies. 25 (2) pp 289–319

Cain, C Surbone, A Elk, R and Kagawa-Singer, M (2018) Culture and palliative care: preferences, communication, meaning and mutual decision making. *Journal of Pain and Symptom Management*, 55(5): 1408–1419.

Care Quality Commission (CQC) (2023) *Experts by Experience*. Available at: www.cqc.org.uk/about-us/jobs/experts-experience (accessed 12 October 2023).

Cohen, L Manion, L and Morrison, K (2018) *Research Methods in Education.* Abingdon: Routledge.

de St Croix, T (2016) *Grassroots Youth Work: Policy, Passion and Resistance in Practice.* Bristol: Policy Press.

Doherty, P Stott, A and Kinder, K (2004) *Delivering Services to Hard-to-Reach Families in On Track Areas: Definition, Consultation and Needs Assessment.* Home Office Development and Practice Report, 15.

Dolmans, D Loyens, S Marcq, H and Gijbels, D (2016) Deep and surface learning in problem-based learning: a review of the literature. *Advances in Health Sciences Education.* 21: 1087–1112.

Dyer, S and Hurd, F (2016) "What's going on?" Developing reflexivity in the management classroom: from surface to deep learning and everything in between. *Academy of Management Learning and Education*, 15(2). https://doi.org/10.5465/amle.2014.0104

Eigenberger, M and Sealander, K (2001) A scale for measuring students' anti-intellectualism. *Psychological Reports*, 89(2): 387–402.

Elander, J Foster, E Norton, L and Foxcroft, A (2010) What changes in the transition to learning at university? In: Rust, C (ed) *Improving Student learning for the 21st Century Learner.* Oxford: Oxfords Centre for Staff and Learning Development, pp 109–124.

Gormally, S and Coburn, A (2014) Finding nexus: connecting youth work and research practices. *British Educational Research Journal*, 40(5): 869–885.

Gravlee, C (2020) Systemic racism, chronic health inequities, and COVID-19: A syndemic in the making? *American Journal of Human Biology*, 32(5): 1–8.

Gregson, M Pollard, A Nixon, L and Spedding, T (2015) *Readings for Reflective Teaching in Further, Adult and Vocational Education.* London: Bloomsbury.

Gyamfi, P (2020) Communication effectiveness: examining interactions between college health professionals and students on university campuses. *Journal of American College Health*, 7(3) https://doi.org/10.1080/07448481.2020.1763367

Hall, S (1990) Cultural identity and diaspora. In: Rutherford, J (ed) *Identity, Community, Culture, Difference.* London: Lawrence and Wishart, pp 222–237.

Hean, S Clark, J Adams, K and Humphris, D (2009) Will opposites attract? Similarities and differences in students' perceptions of the stereotype profiles of other health and social care professional groups. *Journal of Interprofessional Care*, 20(2): 162–181. https://doi.org/10.1080/13561820600646546

Hoi, V (2023) Transitioning from school to university: a person-oriented approach to understanding first-year students' classroom engagement in higher education. *Educational Review.* https://doi-org.ezproxy.derby.ac.uk/10.1080/00131911.2022.2159935

Holmes, A (2020) Researcher positionality – a consideration of its influence and lace in qualitative research – a new researchers guide. *Shanlax International Journal of Education*, 8(4): 1–10. https://doi.org/10.34293/education.v8i4.3232

Horgan, A Manning FO Donovan M Doody R Savage E Bradley S Dorrity C O'Sullivan H Goodwin J Greaney S Biering P Bjornsson Bocking J Russell S MacGabhann L Griffin M van der Vaart K Allon J Granerud A Hals E Pulli J Vatula A Ellila H Lahti M and Happell B (2020) Expert by experience involvement in mental health nursing education: the co-production of standards between experts by experience and academics in mental health nursing. *Journal of Psychiatric and Mental Health Nursing*, 27(5): 555.

Jentleson, B and Ratner, E (2011) Bridging the beltway—ivory tower gap. *International Studies Review,* 13(1): 6–11.

Lepgold, J and Nincic, M (2001) *Beyond the Ivory Tower: International Relations Theory and the Issue of Policy Relevance.* New York: Columbia University Press.

Lochmiller, C and Lester, J (2017) *An Introduction to Educational Research.* London: Sage.

Marmor, J (2006) The felling of superiority: an occupational hazard in the practice of psychotherapy. *The American Journal of Psychiatry*, 110(5): 370–376. https://doi.org/10.1176/ajp.110.5.370

McGinn, T and Burns, P (2023) Coproduction with service users in adult social work: a study of services user' and social workers' experiences in Northern Ireland. *The British Journal of Social Work*: 1–18. https://doi.org/10.1093/bjsw/bcad151

Moss, B (2017) *Communication Skills in Health and Social Care*. London: Sage.

Mulholland, J (2015) Academics: forget about public engagement, stay in your ivory towers. *The Guardian*. Available at: www.theguardian.com/higher-education-network/2015/dec/10/academics-forget-about-public-engagement-stay-in-your-ivory-towers (accessed 3 November 2023).

Nursing Notes (2022) Former Brexit Secretary Steve Barclay appointed as new Health Secretary. Available at https://nursingnotes.co.uk/news/former-brexit-secretary-steve-barclay-appointed-as-new-health-secretary/ (accessed on 28 March 2025).

Nye, J (2008) Bridging the gap between theory and policy. *Political Psychology*, 29(4): 593–603.

Peat, J (2017) These are the top 10 most "pointless degrees". *The London Economic*. Available at: www.thelondoneconomic.com/news/top-10-pointless-degrees-56750/ (accessed 31 September 2023).

Peters, M (2018) Anti-intellectualism is a virus. *Educational Philosophy and Theory*, 51(4): 357–363.

Phillips, F (2021) University degrees can be worthless and leave young people drowning in debt. *Mirror*. Available at: www.mirror.co.uk/news/uk-news/university-not-worth-can-expensive-25331860 (accessed 31 September 2023).

Phillpott, S (2022) The 20 most useless university degrees *CareerAddict*. Available at: www.careeraddict.com/useless-degrees (accessed 31 September 2023)

Ponterotto, J and Grieger, I (2007) Effectively communicating qualitative research. *The Counselling Psychologist*, 35(3): 405–430.

Pritchard, A (2017) *Ways of Learning: Learning Theories for the Classroom*. 4th Edn. London: Routledge.

Purcell, B (2022) Should I be scared when you say that you love me? Youth work practice and power of professional love. In: Dikova, S McMahon, W and Savage, J. (eds) *Love and Politics of Care: Methods, Pedagogies, Institutions*. London: Bloomsbury, pp 149–168.

Racine, L and Vanderberg, H (2021) A philosophical analysis of anti-intellectualism in nursing: Newman's view of a university education. *Nursing Philosophy*, 22(3).

Rawlins, C (2019) The ivory tower of academia and how mental health is often neglected. *Future Science*, 5(4).

Stuart, K Maynard, L and Rouncefield, C (2016) *Evaluation Practice for Projects with Young People*. London: Sage.

Searcey, R (2022) Capturing accidental moments: the self-reflective researcher and the utility of the research diary. In: Sanders, T McGarry, K and Ryan, P (eds) *Sex Work, Labour and Relations*. Cham: Palgrave Macmillan, pp 185–208.

Sunderland, N Stevens, F Knudsen, K Cooper, R and Wobcke, M (2022) Trauma aware and anti-oppressive art-health and community arts practice: guiding principles for facilitating healing, health and wellbeing. *Trauma, Violence and Abuse*, 24(4): 2429–2447 https://doi.org/10.1177/15248380221097442

Thompson, N (2015) *People Skills*. London: Macmillan Education UK.

Thyberg, C (2022) Preparing social workers for anti-oppressive practice: evaluating the role of critical social work education. *Journal of Social Work Education*, 59(2): 407–422. https://doi.org/10.1080/10437797.2022.2119060

Tolsgaard, M Kulasegaram, K Woods, N Brydges, R Ringsted, C and Dyre, L (2020) The myth of ivory tower versus practice-oriented research: a systematic review of randomised studies in medical education. *Medical Education*, 55(3): 328–335. https://doi.org/10.1111/medu.14373

Veldmeijer, L Terlouw, G Van Os, J Van Dijk, O Van't Veer, J and Boonstra, N (2023) The involvement of service users and people with lived experience in mental health care innovation through design. *Systematic Review*, 10. *JMIR Mental Health*: 1–16.

Vygotsky, L S (1978) *Mind in Society: The Development of Higher Psychological Process.* Cambridge MA: Harvard University Press.

Williams, S and Conroy, D (a) (2022) Being prepared. In: Williams, S and Conroy, D (eds) A *Student's guide to Placements in Health and Social Care Settings.* St Albans: Critical Publishing, pp 7–20.

Wood, J Westwood, S and Thompson, G (2014) *Youth Work: Preparation for Practice* London: Routledge.

CHAPTER 2

Introduction to research

Julie Bernstein, Jay Jones, Jessica Millington and Alessia Renganeschi

Introduction

'Bad things happen when problems are protected by a force field of tediousness' (Goldacre, 2011). Anyone about to study research methods rarely jumps for joy, health and social care students being no exception. Why is this, when the importance of evidence-based practice and being consumers of research is dutifully explained, as is the requirement to keep up to date to maintain best practice and, if applicable, registration? It is often still an abstract idea and there are other modules, or life, competing for attention. Learning about practical skills with a more obvious application to professional practice will win the popularity contest every time. The terminology can be impenetrable, adding to the potential dryness of the subject. Yet research is the backbone of health and social care work. It is what underpins and gives credibility to what each profession does, and it changes over time, developing and improving, making it even more important to grasp the concepts at an early stage. Goldacre's quote was referring to the massive amount of data already in existence that was not being utilised to its full extent, but it is also applicable when health and social care professionals do what has always been done, rather than look for the underpinning evidence or test the efficacy of their practice. It is also worth considering that most people do research. Most people have questions, gather information to test their theories, and make decisions based on what they find out. Much formal research follows a similar process to this informal research, for example, when making an expensive purchase. It is likely, therefore, that you come to this topic with some skills.

This chapter is an introduction to health and social care research, looking at it from a historical and professional perspective, and including some of the concepts which will be covered in more detail in subsequent chapters.

DOI: 10.4324/9781041056782-4

Chapter concepts
This chapter addresses the following concepts:

- What is research?
- Lessons from health and social care research history
- Ways we are involved in research
- Keeping your interest

What is research?

Different books and articles will give you varying definitions, depending on the type of research upon which they focus. Social research texts' attention is on the social world and people's interpretations of social phenomena (Clark et al, 2021; May and Perry, 2022). Health sources tend to be more focused on testing theories and the effectiveness of healthcare practice (UK Research and Innovation, 2023). These views may seem incompatible, but health and social care work is with human beings who live in the social world but also need this work to be the best possible, using the most effective interventions. Moreover, there is no point in advising a course of action if there are barriers to people being able to make a choice to engage. Therefore, it is as useful to find out the impact of a situation on someone and the impact of our work with them, as the work itself, to maximise concordance.

This debate about definition also relates to the underlying philosophical concepts and beliefs about knowledge: what truth or truths there are to learn and how we may learn them (in research terminology this is referred to as ontology and epistemology) (Benton and Craib, 2023). Bowling (2023, p 1), however, gives the following definition that: 'research is the systematic and rigorous process of enquiry which aims to describe phenomena and to develop and test explanatory concepts and theories' combining the two viewpoints. Additionally, the National Institute for Health and Care Research (NIHR, no date) gives a specific definition about social care research focusing 'on the evidence needed to improve people's wellbeing and independence, protect human rights and promote equality'. Therefore, people new to research need to consider that there are multiple definitions of what research is, and to consider their own situation and context.

Lessons from health and social care research history

Although people have been seeking remedies for illness and better quality of life for as long as there have been people in existence, evidence of research as we think of it now is harder to find. In ancient Mesopotamia, texts of a medical nature exist, alongside archaeology, but some of the words are untranslatable and it is surmised that because the remedies had been used for centuries, they must have worked (Zucconi and Moss, 2019). Jumping forward to the 1800s in colonial North America, herbal remedies were favoured by African American healers. This was a complex process, passed down by apprenticeship, so that different plants could be identified safely, along with a wealth of other skills (Fett, 2002). This was both mocked and appropriated by white patriarchal European colonisers, thereby whitewashing representation of those who pioneered great leaps in health and care innovation (Baker and Wynia, 2021; Dominus, 2019). Nowadays, commissioners of health and social care services will not be impressed even by experienced professionals telling them that they do what they always did because it works, as alluded to earlier. Therefore, the rest of this section will consider a selection of the improvements in health and social care research that have contributed to current practice, starting with Table 2.1 highlighting some pioneers of practice.

Table 2.1 Selected pioneers in health and social care research

Name	Dates lived	Expertise	Breakthrough	Reference/s
Andreas Vesalius	1514–1546	Human dissection	Disproved works of Galen. Published drawings.	Hepburn and Anderson (2021) Wootton (2006) Zampieri et al (2015)
John Snow	1813–1858	Physician in multiple fields	'Father of public health' Tracked cholera, proving a source, contributing to creation of germ theory.	Begum (2016) Wootton (2006)
James McCune Smith	1813–1865	Physician	First African American to earn a medical degree.	Brown (2024) Kreuter et al (2021) Lujan and DiCarlo (2019) Morgan (2003) Smith (1846 & 1859)
Florence Nightingale	1820–1910	Nurse	Cleanliness and Epidemiology – publishing statistical information on circumstances of deaths.	Downs (2023) McDonald (2004) Tulchinsky (2018) Wootton (2006)
Jane Addams	1860–1935	Social Worker	First American woman awarded Nobel Peace Prize. Participatory research, involving advocacy.	Beames et al (2021) Shields (2017)
Mildred Blaxter	1925–2010	Social researcher	Meaning of disability. Intergenerational health and social inequality and deprivation. Central to the first national survey of health and lifestyles.	Corti-Georgiou (2019) Thompson (2019a) Thompson (2019b)
Stuart Hall	1932–2014	Social researcher/ academic	A creator of Cultural Studies and new interpretative approaches for analysis of popular culture.	UK Data Service (2018)

Although not a pioneer in dissection itself, which already had a long history (Hepburn and Anderson, 2021; Wootton, 2006), Andreas Vesalius was able to combine the study of anatomy with drawings, enabling others to learn from what he had achieved and assisted by improvements in the ability to print books (Zampieri et al, 2015). This was a massive step forward from the previously mentioned apprenticeship model of passing down information by word of mouth, enabling good practice to be documented and shared. John Snow and Florence Nightingale also developed what is now established as epidemiology (or the study of population health), using observation, recording of numbers, and circumstances of deaths to improve mortality rates by various means (Downs, 2023; Tulchinsky, 2018; Wootton, 2006). Snow is celebrated as the founding father of public health and modern epidemiology, but there are assertions that the origins of epidemiology were in the exploitation of African slaves, and it is important to remember there were those who had no agency to tell their own stories. 'Modern epidemiological practices grew in part out of observing, treating, and preventing disease among captive populations produced by colonialism, slavery, and war' (Downs, 2023, p 197). The countries Nightingale travelled to and the amount of statistical information in her public health works is staggering, but it is also argued that this contributed to seeing native people in the colonies as numbers rather than human beings (McDonald, 2004; Downs, 2023). We therefore need to be mindful of learning lessons regarding respect for human beings who are research participants, not just treating research ethics as a tick-box exercise, and being actively anti-oppressive.

Although earning his qualifications, James McCune Smith's research faced barriers on publication. Despite authoring the first ever case report written by a black physician, he was stopped from presenting this to the New York Medical and Surgery Society, due to fears of upsetting the 'harmony' of the institution (Morgan, 2003; Smith, 1859). In his publication "A Dissertation on the Influence of Climate on Longevity" (1846), Smith's use of statistical analysis and advanced statistical methods highlighted that the health outcomes of black people within the slave trade were not comparable to 'free' black men and women (Lujan and DiCarlo, 2019). Smith's work was influential in addressing racial health inequalities within America and his story exemplifies the power that the research process can have in addressing inequalities, but also acts as a hard reminder that barriers did, and still do, exist within health and social care research (Kreuter et al, 2021). By reflecting on Smith's story, it is ever important to remember that research should be diverse, equitable, accessible, and, where appropriate, grounded by the experiences of underrepresented communities.

Social research has as much importance for health and social care professionals as health research, in that you and those you work with are all involved in the social world; you rely on communication and are affected by the structures and belief systems that human beings have created (Clark et al, 2021). Jane Addams, a pioneering social worker and feminist, focused on participatory research, providing many lessons worthwhile considering when approaching research methods today. Her devotion to community involvement, engagement, and collaboration in social research highlights the importance of qualitative research and its ability to produce relevant and actionable data (Beames et al, 2021). Addams' approach to empirical research served as a basis for her advocacy in social policy and reform. A key lesson that her story teaches is that research is more powerful when coupled with advocacy. Her research was used as a tool for change and that acts as a reminder of its important role in health and social reform.

There is large repository of life story interviews with important social researchers freely available, diverse in gender and ethnicity, and with global locations of their research entitled 'Pioneers of Qualitative Research' and located in the UK Data Service repository (Corti-Georgiou, 2019; Thompson, 2019a; UK Data Service, 2018). Within this archive can be found an interview with Mildred Blaxter, a social researcher, who began her career before qualitative methodologies had '*solidified*' (Thompson, 2019b, para 192). Her most pivotal research was in medical welfare, the meaning of disability and latterly a study on health and illness in a sample of women born prior to the start of the NHS. This demonstrated that deprivation continued across generations due to poverty and inequality, rather than any fault of the people concerned. Another social researcher in this archive is Stuart Hall, who, Jamaican by birth, moved to Britain both to escape the colonialism of his surroundings and to study. He became pivotal in creating the field of cultural studies. Within this he included issues of race and gender and developed new interpretative approaches for analysis of popular culture and its influence (UK Data Service, 2018). The creation of new intersectional areas of research interest and study are as important for health and social care practitioners' development as they are on the development of new ways to conduct research. A diverse variety of viewpoints need appreciation as well as all the influences and determinants on health and well-being, otherwise research will continue to marginalise oppressed groups of people and lessons hard learnt from history will have been wasted.

It is therefore important in your learning about and involvement with research that you endeavour to be inclusive, recognise your position of power, and respect the need for ethical approval, not seeking to circumvent it; all of which you will find more about in chapters 1 (Power in research), 4 (Ethical considerations in health and social care research), 7 (Including vulnerable participants in research), and 8 (Involvement of people with lived experiences in research).

How we are involved in research

One way health and social care practitioners are involved in research is keeping practice up to date by reading, and attending training and conferences (Health and Care Professions Council [HCPC], 2024; Nursing and Midwifery Council, 2021). An extension of this is evidence-based practice, whereby you both improve what you do and justify it to everyone, from service users to commissioners (Heaslip and Lindsay, 2019). This is why student practitioners are taught the skills to locate evidence that proves what they do works, including assessments, one to one and group interventions, outcome measures and more. This is often by reading, but you also need to judge if what you read is trustworthy and applicable to your work, in other words, critical appraisal (Aveyard et al, 2015; Aveyard et al, 2022). Not only do you need to justify your current practice, but you may also need to find a new solution by seeking research evidence, which may then require translation into your setting.

Applying the research methodologies and practice that you have read about to your practice is valid to conducting research. After all, research is pointless without application. Journal clubs are one way to support each other in keeping up to date, appraising research relevant to your practice and working out how it can be applied (Deenadaya-lan et al, 2008). In a typical journal club, a member chooses a research article, everyone reads it, and then the group discusses its quality and relevance to practice. It is important to document a journal club for your continuing professional development portfolio as evidence of continuous learning and staying up to date, both to meet professional body standards (HCPC, 2024) and for your own ethical satisfaction that you are doing the best you can for those with whom you work. Peer review also plays a vital role in research. Evaluating and providing feedback on articles submitted for publication in academic journals or on conference abstracts enhances the quality of the publication and the presentation. By engaging in these activities, practitioners actively contribute to the advancement of their field and improve their practice through research.

Practitioners can also participate in empirical research, which may involve recruiting participants (e.g. service users), collecting data for others' research using outcome measures, or conducting research independently. For example, if you create a questionnaire to evaluate a group intervention, this is research. It does not have to be a complicated piece of experimental research, although health and social care practitioners do also work as researchers, carrying out primary and secondary research.

It is crucial to recognise that all research must adhere to strict ethical standards, which will be discussed further in Chapter 4. In any research involving the recruitment of participants, researchers have an ethical duty of care to protect and uphold the dignity and rights of those involved. This includes ensuring informed consent, protecting confidentiality, and guarding against any potential harm to participants. Additionally, the data collected must be managed with transparency and integrity, ensuring it is obtained and stored legally.

Keeping your interest
It is helpful to be aware of your learning needs, preferred ways to learn, and the resources available to you. There is a wealth of valid information about research beyond books and articles, such as videos on the internet, but there needs to be discernment about the quality. Various lengths of film and audio recordings on all aspects of research can be found (see Table 2.2 for recommended resources). The point to remember is to use these resources to help understand the concepts, but to then return to the reference books and academic articles to use as supporting references in assignments. This is because of the quality control processes in research articles coming to publication, such as peer review, making them more credible. Nevertheless, online videos, radio programmes, podcasts, and audiobooks can make this subject more accessible and memorable.

Completing surveys emailed from other students, satisfaction surveys, and market research gives insight into how particular questions make you feel. Sometimes you must be tenacious to be a participant in other people's research because they have not thought through the participant experience (Boyd et al, 2024). This gives you valuable insight for when it is your turn. Afterall, without participants you do not have any research (if your research involves people), therefore you need to make it as easy as possible for them to take part.

There are books which can help you see the point of evidence-based practice and research in a light-hearted way (see Table 2.2). There are also a multitude of critical appraisal checklists and books. The idea is that you learn how research is ideally

Table 2.2 Recommended resources

Resource type	Name	Where to find it
Video	TED Talks	See TED (2011, 2012, 2017)
Audio	The Infinite Monkey Cage	www.bbc.co.uk/programmes/b00snr0w
Audio	More or Less	www.bbc.co.uk/programmes/b006qshd
Audio	Thinking Allowed	www.bbc.co.uk/programmes/b006qy05
Book	*Bad Science* by Ben Goldacre	Goldacre (2009)
Book	Bad Medicine by Ian Wootton	Wootton (2006)
Book	*How to Read a Paper* by Trisha Greenhalgh	Greenhalgh (2019)
Book	*The Pocket Guide to Critical Appraisal* by Iain Crombie	Crombie (2022)
Online Resource	Critical Skills Appraisal Programme	http://casp-uk.net/casp-tools-checklists/
Book	*Research Methods in Health: Investigating Health and Health Services* by Ann Bowling	Bowling (2023)
Book and online resource	*Bryman's Social Research Methods* by Clark et al	Clark et al (2021)
Book	*The Good Research Guide* by Martyn Denscombe	Denscombe (2021)

carried out so you can systematically appraise articles without treating them differently, for example, not being harder on qualitative research because you prefer quantitative. It is worth developing a curious, questioning, critical eye for everything you read (Aveyard et al, 2015). Not all items in a checklist, even if dedicated to the specific type of research you are appraising, will apply to all articles of that type. It can take some confidence to write 'not applicable' on your checklist. This is where checking out the alternatives, such as books on critical appraisal, can be helpful, as some are easier to comprehend than others. There are also multiple options for general research texts that cover a wide range of information at a basic level. Choose the one that you prefer, perhaps one that includes a good glossary to help with the terminology.

If studying at a more advanced level, you will need to delve further into specific methodologies. There will be respected theorists whose work you need to know and an expectation that you will use more literature from academic journals (Wette, 2021), but you can also find alternative literature and multimedia resources that help you to understand these tomes. You have choices, but you need to do enough reading to appreciate and justify your choices. How you reach that point is up to you.

Student voice
READ! Research texts are full of alien terminology which at first sight can be incredibly daunting. Gain an understanding of what these terms mean, as this sets the foundation for understanding research methods. Don't panic, terminology takes time to learn, and creating a glossary of definitions supports your understanding. Also, critically appraising articles continues throughout your research journey; and lastly, allow time to really understand the intricacies of research methods and the research process. – Jay

My advice is to step into research being as open-minded as possible. This is particularly true when approaching a research topic about which you already have a passion or opinion. I would advise other students to acknowledge their bias rather than labelling it as negative, as it adds value to their research perspective, and to understand and engage in activities such as reflexivity, because that is the moment in which their bias can lead to additional value. Practically speaking, keep a research diary, being as honest and transparent as possible about the reasons underlying the research. After all, the biggest discovery is the one we know nothing about – yet. – Alessia

I would highlight the significance of curiosity, critical thinking, and organisation. Begin by selecting a topic that genuinely interests you, as this will fuel your motivation throughout the research journey. Once a topic area has been decided, I would emphasise the importance of conducting a thorough literature search to be aware of existing knowledge and identify gaps in research. Remember to scrutinise sources for credibility and relevance, establishing a strong foundation for your work. Also, don't forget librarians, who are excellent at providing advice and support. Finally, embrace the iterative nature of research, be prepared to revise and refine your work as you uncover new information, often the question you begin with might not be where you end up. Always approach research with an open mind, a systematic approach, and a willingness to learn from the process.

Conclusion

In this chapter, several aspects have been discussed to start answering why, as health and social care professionals, research in these fields represents an important aspect of your practice. Research is critical for evidence-based practice in health and social care. While it may seem abstract and less appealing compared to practical skills, it underpins the credibility of the profession by continuously improving practices.

If you were thinking about research as something distant from you, now you may have considered a different perspective, appreciating that everyone engages in informal research in everyday life. Formal research in health and social care (and other disciplines as well) follows similar processes, involving inquiry, data gathering, and decision-making based on evidence. While in health, research often focuses on testing theories and the effectiveness of interventions, in social research there is more focus on understanding social phenomena and the impact of the social world. Despite these differences, both perspectives are vital as health and social care professionals work within social contexts. As future health and social care professionals, you are likely to be or become involved in research in multiple ways, including staying updated with current evidence, participating in journal clubs, peer reviews, and even conducting your own empirical research.

The concept of research and its connection to ontology (what can be known) and epistemology (how we come to know it), and therefore to the larger generative process that leads to new knowledge, have been discussed. Due to its complexity, multiple definitions of research exist, depending on context and discipline. However, a brief historical overview highlights key pioneers in health and social care research, giving recognition to the evolution of research methods and the need to be both critical and inclusive in the practice of research.

Talking about research or becoming more directly involved in it may feel intimidating, and staying motivated can be a significant challenge. However, in this chapter you will have found that research does not need to be done in one way only. Knowing your learning preferences and exploring various multimedia formats can make research more accessible and engaging for you. You are encouraged to be curious, not only about the topic of research, but also about you as a researcher. Critical thinking and curiosity are essential in navigating research. Common themes from the student advice given are to keep an open mind, identify your own interests and biases, and to be critical in all aspects of the research process. They also emphasise the importance of thorough literature searches, critical appraisal of sources, and being flexible in the research process.

To conclude, in this chapter it has been emphasised how research is fundamental to improving health and social care practices, and while it can seem daunting when you are approaching it as a student, there are many resources and approaches to make it more engaging and applicable to real-world practice.

Reflective questions

1. What are your initial feelings about research?
2. Where do these feelings come from?
3. What might help you engage with learning about research?

References

Aveyard, H Preston, N and Farquhar, M (2022) *How to Read and Critique Research: A Guide for Nursing and Healthcare Students*. London: SAGE.

Aveyard, H Sharp, P and Woolliams, M (2015) *Critical Thinking and Writing in Health and Social Care*. 2nd Edn. Maidenhead: Open University Press.

Baker, R and Wynia, M (2021) Living histories of structural racism and organized medicine. *AMA Journal of Ethics*, 23(12): 995–1003.

Beames, JR Kikas, K O'Gradey-Lee, M Gale, N Werner-Seidler, A Boydell, KM and Hudson, JL (2021) A new normal: integrating lived experience into scientific data syntheses. *Frontiers in Psychiatry*, 12: 763005.

Begum, F (2016) *Mapping Disease: John Snow and Cholera*. Available at: www.rcseng.ac.uk/library-and-publications/library/blog/mapping-disease-john-snow-and-cholera/ (accessed on 31 March 2025).

Benton, T and Craib, I (2023) *Philosophy of Social Science*. 3rd Edn. London: Bloomsbury Publishing.

Boyd, P Sternke, E Tite, D and Morgan, K (2024) There was no opportunity to express good or bad: perspectives from patient focus groups on patient experience in clinical trials. *Journal of Patient Experience*, 11: 1–6.

Bowling, A (2023) *Research Methods in Health: Investigating Health and Health Services*. 5th Edn. Maidenhead: Open University Press.

Brown, J (2024) The battle to become a Black physician in the USA: past and present. *The Lancet*, 403(10425): 426–428.

Clark, T Foster, L Sloan, S and Bryman, A (2021) *Bryman's Social Research Methods*. 6th Edn. Oxford: Oxford University Press.

Corti-Georgiou, C (2019) Pioneers of social research: a life story interview collection. *Research Data Journal for the Humanities and Social Sciences,* 4(1): 91–108.

Crombie, I (2022) *The Pocket Guide to Critical Appraisal*. 2nd Edn. Chichester: Wiley-Blackwell.

Deenadayalan, Y Grimmer-Somers, K, Prior, M and Kumar S (2008) How to run an effective journal club: a systematic review. *Journal of Evaluation in Clinical Practice*, 14(5): 898–911.

Denscombe, M (2021) *The Good Research Guide*. 7th Edn. Maidenhead: Open University Press.

Dominus, S (2019) Women scientists were written out of history. *Smithsonian Magazine*, October. Available at: www.smithsonianmag.com/science-nature/unheralded-women-scientists-finally-getting-their-due-180973082/ (accessed 29 November 2024).

Downs, J (2023) *Maladies of Empire: How Colonialism, Slavery, and War Transformed Medicine*. London: The Belknap Press of Harvard University Press.

Fett, S (2002) *Working Cures: Healing, Health and Power on Southern Slave Plantations*. Chapel Hill: University of North Caroline Press.

Goldacre, B (2009) *Bad Science*. London: Fourth Estate.

Goldacre, B (2011) There's a wealth of data out there – why not let us use it? *The Guardian*, 7 October. Available at: www.theguardian.com/commentisfree/2011/oct/07/wealth-of-data-locked-away (accessed 29 November 2024).

Greenhalgh, T (2019) *How to Read a Paper*. 6th Edn. Chichester: Wiley-Blackwell.

Heaslip, V and Lindsay, B (2019) *Research and Evidence-Based Practice*. Banbury: Lantern Publishing Ltd.

Health and Care Professions Council (HCPC) (2024) *What is CPD?* Available at: www.hcpc-uk.org/cpd/our-cpd-requirements/ (accessed 29 November 2024).

Hepburn, B and Anderson, H (2021) Scientific method. *The Stanford Encyclopaedia of Philosophy*. Available at: https://plato.stanford.edu/archives/sum2021/entries/scientific-method/ (accessed 29 November 2024).

Kreuter, MW Thompson, T McQueen, A and Garg, R (2021) Addressing social needs in health care settings: evidence, challenges, and opportunities for public health. *Annual Review of Public Health*, 42: 329–344.

Lujan, HL and DiCarlo, SE (2019) First African American to hold a medical degree: brief history of James McCune Smith, abolitionist, educator, and physician. *Advances in Physiology Education*, 43(2): 134–139.

May, T and Perry, B (2022) *Social Research: Issues, Methods and Processes*. 5th Edn. Maidenhead: Open University Press.

McDonald, L, (Ed) (2004) *Florence Nightingale on Public Health Care. Volume 6 of the Collected Works of Florence Nightingale*. Ontario: Wilfred Laurier University Press.

Morgan, TM (2003) The education and medical practice of Dr James McCune Smith (1813–1865), first black American to hold a medical degree. *Journal of the National Medical Association*, 95(7): 603–614.

National Institute for Health and Care Research (NIHR) (no date) *What is Health and Care Research*. Available at: https://bepartofresearch.nihr.ac.uk/what-is-health-and-care-research/#:~:text=Social%20care%20research%20is%20about,human%20rights%20and%20promote%20equality (accessed 29 November 2024).

Nursing and Midwifery Council (2021) *Continuing Professional Development*. Available at: www.nmc.org.uk/revalidation/requirements/cpd/ (accessed 29 November 2024).

Shields, P (2017) *Jane Addams: Progressive Pioneer of Peace, Philosophy, Sociology, Social Work and Public Administration: 10*. New York: Springer.

Smith, JM (1846) A dissertation on the influence of climate on longevity. *Journal of the National Medical Association*.

Smith, JM (1859) Chess. *The Anglo-African Magazine*, September: 273–278.

TED (2011) *Ben Goldacre: Battling Bad Science*. July 2011. Available at: www.ted.com/talks/ben_goldacre_battling_bad_science?subtitle=en (accessed 29 November 2024).

TED (2012) *Ben Goldacre: What Doctors Don't Know About the Drugs They Prescribe*. July. Available at: www.ted.com/talks/ben_goldacre_what_doctors_don_t_know_about_the_drugs_they_prescribe?subtitle=en (accessed 29 November 2024).

TED (2017) *Mona Chalabi: 3 Ways to Spot a Bad Statistic.* February. Available at: www.ted.com/talks/mona_chalabi_3_ways_to_spot_a_bad_statistic?subtitle=en (accessed 29 November 2024).

Thompson, P (2019a) *Pioneers of Social Research: 1995–2018.* [data collection] 4th Edn. UK Data Service. SN: 6226, DOI: doi.org/10.5255/UKDA-SN-6226-6.

Thompson, P (2019b) *University of Essex, Department of Sociology: Interview with Mildred Blaxter, in "Pioneers of Social Research, 1996–2018".* 4th Edn, Para. 192. Available at: https://discover.ukdataservice.ac.uk/QualiBank/Document/?cid=q-e8a26642-ca19-42b5-be4a-1fa25763b6ac (accessed 29 November 2024).

Tulchinsky, T (2018) *Case Studies in Public Health.* Massachusetts: Elsevier Science and Technology.

UK Data Service (2018) *Bio-Bibliographical Guide Pioneers of Social Research.* Available at: https://ukdataservice.ac.uk/learning-hub/qualitative-data/#pioneers-of-qualitative-research (accessed 29 November 2024).

UK Research and Innovation (2023) *Understanding Health Research.* Available at: www.ukri.org/councils/mrc/facilities-and-resources/find-an-mrc-facility-or-resource/mrc-regulatory-support-centre/understanding-health-research/what-is-health-research/ (accessed 29 November 2024).

Wette, R (2021) *Writing Using Sources for Academic Purposes: Theory, Research and Practice.* London: Routledge.

Wootton, D (2006) *Bad Medicine.* Oxford: Oxford University Press.

Zampieri, F ElMaghawry, M Zanatta, A and Thiene, G (2015) Andreas Vesalius: celebrating 500 years of dissecting nature. *Global Cardiology Science and Practice,* (5): 66.

Zucconi, L and Moss, C (2019) *Ancient Medicine: From Mesopotamia to Rome.* Chicago: William B. Eerdmans Publishing Company.

Importance of research in practice

Michael Balkow, Dolapo Fakuade and Helen Turrell

Introduction

This chapter emphasises the importance of research in health and social care practice, engaging in critical discussion and debates about the benefits, difficulties, and contentions within research. We discuss the everyday nature of research and its connection with practice and the people it is intended to benefit. Research opens the door to knowledge, but the extent can also be overwhelming. Practitioners and students need to interpret, apply, and action research through a critical lens. Research can help guide decision-making with individuals, but it can also illuminate broader areas of society, deepening our knowledge and understanding of areas and elements that affect the population. We draw upon events, such as the Covid-19 pandemic, to locate this chapter within broader global events that impact entire populations. This pandemic accelerated research, especially in finding a safe vaccine and exploration of the impact of lockdowns on wellness and wellbeing. It is important to understand how real-life events may inform research, which may subsequently inform practice to address challenges of dealing with real-life events.

Chapter concepts

- To understand the importance of research in day-to-day practice.
- To explore the benefits, difficulties, and contentions in applying research to everyday practice.

When we talk about the everyday nature of research in this chapter, we are discussing how practitioners can apply research to their practice, and how it would be largely impossible to practice without any prior knowledge of the subject or engaging with researchers who have helped shape the profession. Tied to this are ethical and practice requirement to keep your knowledge and skills up to date, as stipulated by regulating bodies, which is also good ethical practice (see Chapter 4). As Moule (2015, p 3)

DOI: 10.4324/9781041056782-5

states: 'The care provided by all health and social care practitioners must be based on current knowledge and evidence that promotes the delivery of the highest standards of care possible'. Research is not free from difficulty or contention. In order to make it part of the *'everyday'* we need to combine the sometimes-distant worlds of scientific laboratories, universities, and libraries where such knowledge is researched, published, and accessed by students and academics and transposed to health and social care practitioners – touching the lives of the very people and communities it was intended to reach.

Students and practitioners may feel that research is in some ways 'cold and impersonal' (D'Cruz and Jones, 2014, p 2), at odds with the empathetic supporting nature of health and social care, detached from the human connections these professions nurture. Finding and identifying relevant research can also be a challenge, and students would not be alone in this quest, as Belcher (2019, p 186) explores in her guide to writing, that reading the literature (in preparation for writing) is like entering a forest of no return. The more we read, the more we find there is to read about a topic and the reader may become overwhelmed. Therefore, some groundwork preparation may be required, such as accessing guides on research in health and social care, and making use of glossaries that explain research in simple terms (Heaslip and Lindsay, 2019). It is important for students to understand how research can be made more accessible, applicable, and understood to ultimately drive health and social care practice which highlights the application of personal values in research.

Personal values and research

Thompson's Personal, Cultural, and Structural (PCS) model (2020, p 36) is a three-level model that was designed to explore how discrimination can affect people and society, however it can be applied to explain how research may be influenced by different factors or elements. This model can be used by health and social care professionals and students to enable them to develop a clearer understanding of the importance of research, and how research can be understood both in the day-to-day practice and in the wider context of health and social care practice. The first level, Personal (P), refers to the thoughts, feelings, attitudes, and behaviours of individuals and Thompson's model can be applied to show that these behaviours may demonstrate a lack of knowledge or research experience in practice. However, this model could suggest that the broader context in which a practitioner is located could impact on their limited access to research knowledge. For example, practitioners based on hospital wards may not have immediate access to research resources in comparison to university students, or the practitioner may receive a lack of support from management or peers in their setting.

The second level in the PCS model is the Cultural (C) level, which explains that while we have our own individual thoughts, feelings, attitudes, and behaviours, these need to be understood within the wider cultural context. Where there are shared values and norms among practitioners, students, and academics on understanding the potential benefits, outcomes, and positive impacts of undertaking and utilising research knowledge, this may then lead to an increase in positive feelings and attitudes towards research and improved communication amongst students, practitioners, and academics.

Thompson's third Structural (S) level explains how wider societal structures and institutions influence thoughts, feelings, and behaviours. Structural aspects have been shown to influence research in health and social care services which are currently under significant pressure. There is a record demand for services, and an ageing population, resulting in substantial waiting lists, resulting in more health and social care services struggling financially (Powell et al, 2024). These factors impact research because institutions may contribute less to funding research projects as there is less money available. Furthermore, because the demand for health and social care services is higher, practitioners will have less time to conduct research and potentially less support to do so, as their role will fall on colleagues. Bureaucracy is also another element that may be driven by structural aspects. The final report into the independent review of research bureaucracy (Department for Science, Innovation and Technology, 2021) highlighted a lack of trust, partnership working, coordination, and knowledge exchange throughout the sector. Furthermore, the success rate for research grant applications was extremely low at around 20%, affirming the need for change within research.

Personal, Cultural, and Structural aspects explained through the PCS model may be used by students and practitioners alike to identify, understand, and critique evidence from research. While elements of this model are relatable, there are also explanations of how research may influence practice or be perceived by service users which are explained further. Stephen Webb (2001) has provided a critique of how workers use evidence from research in their practice. He sees workers as agents of change who carry an impulse to reform various conditions of service user's live, making decisions not just on evidence, but by incorporating predictions of future harm or wellbeing based on their own value base and professional knowledge. If research takes the worker down one route, yet the client and worker both favour a differing route, the evidence hierarchy may be discounted or altered for more client favourable methods. Webb also views decisions made by workers as falling under the impetus of 'common sense' due to workers operating in spaces of contingency, drawing on inclinations and values (Webb, 2001, p 67). Citing the philosopher Antonio Gramsci, Garrett explains common sense as 'furnishing a blurred, hazy and defective lens through which to view the world because it includes information and forms of reasoning which are objectively inaccurate or crucially incomplete' (Garrett, 2023, pp 599–600). This less sympathetic take on common sense in decision-making broadly highlights some of the fallibility of reasoning from common sense, and the importance of research evidence within practice. Practitioners can use their common sense to determine what should happen in a particular situation, but research needs to inform this. This could involve sourcing research that supports the common-sense conclusion, or also importantly, using research that may contradict or challenge the student or practitioner's assumptions and own conclusions.

It may be a daunting thought that newly qualified practitioners must carry around with them a mental file of up-to-date research and evidence, a type of doctor's satchel that can be drawn from to find the correct treatment, tool, or intervention. Taking the approach from the links between theory and practice, Stepney and Thompson (2021, p 149) reverse the idea that theory should precede practice and instead propose 'theorising practice.' This approach takes its starting point from real-life situations that require a response, then afterwards theorising the practice by working out what elements of a professional's knowledge base will be relevant for the situation.

Retrospection and reflective practice could here be used to identify the research and evidence required, to meet the specific circumstance from an element of practice such as a completed home visit.

Whilst the primary function of research is to provide practitioners with a solid evidence base to facilitate decisions to enhance care, it can also be a way of connecting with people who use the services. Beresford (in Hulatt and Lowes, 2005, p 6) discusses user involvement in research and health and social care policy and practice (see Chapter 11), highlighting the strong and growing interest in user involvement in policy and planning since the 1980s. However, he identifies this has been slower to develop into user involvement in health and social care research. This suggests a certain distance between the primacy of research to the very people it is designed to support and benefit. There is a risk with this disconnect, that research becomes something that is *done* to people rather than *for* the people it supports. Service user movements can generate powers of knowledge production and emancipation (see Chapter 14). For example, the Union of the Physically Impaired Against Segregation (UPIAS), a UK disability rights organisation active in the 1970s, whose radical approach turned the tables on disability from a personal state to a phenomenon created by society's restrictions, imparted upon those with disabilities: 'In our view, it is society which disables physically impaired people. Disability is something imposed on top of our impairments, by the way we are unnecessarily isolated and excluded from full participation in society' (UPIAS in Shakespeare, 2006, p 215).

These radical ideas gave rise to the social model of disability, which sees people with disabilities not being limited by their disabilities on an individual level, but by the society they live in, its barriers, restrictions, and discrimination placed upon them. This was arguably a precursor to the Disability Discrimination Act (1995 c.50), later to be reaffirmed and enshrined into the Equality Act (2010 c.15). There is also a connection to be made here with Participatory Action Research (Lawson et al, 2015), which is an investigative methodology that enables democratic participation in real-word problem solving by local stakeholders. These stakeholders may lack formal research training when the research begins, however will have expertise in problem solving at the local level, making them participants of the research, but also those that stand to benefit from it.

The recent Cass review (2024), an independent review of gender identity services for children and young people, is a recent illustration of how research and evidence can be subject to change and scrutiny, the controversies surrounding the mental health of children, the transgender community and associated toxic debates that go against the principles of supporting societies most vulnerable. One of the report's findings was that puberty blockers only have clearly defined benefits in quite narrow circumstances, with potential risks to neurocognitive development, psychosexual development, and longer-term bone health, therefore concluding that they should only be offered under a research protocol (Cass, 2024). Although this may reduce the mentioned risks, it could also lead young people with gender dysphoria to having limited options, relying heavily on mental health services such as CAMHS, which often have very long waiting lists. A report from the Royal College of Nursing and Public Health England (Public Health England, 2015) summarised research of transgender young people showing that a number of studies suggest they are at a higher risk of depression, self-harm, substance misuse, suicidal thoughts and behaviour, and suicide attempts than cisgender people (see Chapter 7). Although this report is now less recent, with an ex-Conservative politician stating prior to the 2024 general election that it needed to be fought on a mix of culture wars and trans debates (Perry, 2023), thereby exploiting vulnerable groups for political gain, it is unlikely that the situation for transgender people will be one of improvement. Therefore, students and practitioners should keep their knowledge of larger political and societal issues that influence research and policy up to date.

Research informed policy and professional practice

Evidence from health and social care research indicates that research influences, and often shapes, professional practice (Smith et al, 2019). Nyström et al (2018) highlight the importance of collaborative and partnership research, especially when challenging health and social care issues. They identified cooperative research as beneficial to improving services through the transfer of knowledge gained practice.

More studies in Sweden reiterate the central role evidence and research play in health practice and policymaking (Nyström et al, 2018; Strehlenert et al, 2015). Meanwhile Byrne (2012) promotes research findings that reflect the robustness of the research evidence.

Nyström et al (2018) advocate for collaborative approaches to ensure research informs practice. For example, students can collaborate with service users to better understand what is needed, thus developing research aims and questions to ensure that research is impactful (see Chapter 8). It is important to support students to collaborate with service users to achieve the intended outcome of a research, as well as facilitate students' engagement with practitioners to share findings from their research. By incorporating evidence-based approaches, practitioners can ensure they deliver high-quality, equitable services that meet the diverse needs of individuals accessing health and social care services. Research-informed policy and professional practice are fundamental to adequate health and social care provision (Strehlenert et al, 2015). The Covid-19 pandemic underscored the critical role of research in guiding health and social care practices, highlighting the importance of evidence-based decision-making in addressing a public health crisis. Though not without its challenges, evidence-based decision-making may not necessarily produce similar policies in similar circumstances or lead to better lessons learned between context (Rubin et al, 2021). By integrating evidence from research, theory, and law into professional practice, practitioners can ensure that they deliver high-quality, equitable services that meet the diverse needs of individuals accessing health and social care services. However, it is acknowledged that evidence-based decision-making may not sufficiently address all issues pertaining to health and social care services due to uncertainties emanating from evolving situations (Lancaster et al, 2020). While such uncertainties might act as barriers, students are in a good position to explore how their research might inform practice.

Studies conducted during the Covid-19 pandemic, examining the effects of social isolation and loneliness on mental health, have underscored the importance of maintaining social connections, even amidst physical distancing measures (Holmes et al, 2020). Health and social care practitioners have adapted their approaches to provide support remotely, utilising technology to facilitate virtual interactions and deliver essential services to vulnerable populations (Rajan et al, 2020). This demonstrates how research can influence practice; an example students may reference and be motivated by in their career path. Furthermore, research into the virus's transmission, symptoms, and potential treatments has been pivotal in guiding healthcare professionals' response to the pandemic. For instance, the World Health Organization (WHO) conducted studies in 2020 on the efficacy of various vaccines and treatments which have informed vaccination strategies and clinical protocols across the world. Similarly, research by the Centers for Disease Control and Prevention (CDC) in the United States of America (USA) on public health interventions shaped the practice. During Covid-19, the CDC research in 2020 on mask-wearing and social distancing shaped government policies to control the spread of the virus. This shows the potential of research to directly inform practice, policy, and public behaviour to mitigate health risks.

Reflective question

Using the experience of Covid-19, can students reflect how they could approach research by investigating other health risks that can benefit from further research in order to mitigate such health risks?

Students can be motivated by this positive evidence from Covid-19, which reflects the power in research and the potential impact on the public (see Chapter 14). As explained earlier in this chapter, students can achieve positive impact with their research by collaborating with service users. Thus, it is pertinent for students to reflect how they might collaborate with service users to understand public behaviour in relation to health risk to determine appropriate mitigation measures or practices.

Prior to, during, and post pandemic era, evidence of how research informs practice abounds, but also is its influence on policy. Research-informed policy shapes the broader health and social care systems. In most countries, including the UK, there is expectation from healthcare policymakers to develop evidence-based policies which are generated by researchers (Gabbay et al, 2020). Policy decisions informed by robust research evidence are more likely to address populations' needs and promote health equity effectively. For example, research highlighting disparities in access to healthcare services among marginalized communities can inform policy interventions to reduce health inequalities (Marmot et al, 2020). This example highlights how students might ensure their research is impactful. It is reassuring to students to know that by identifying healthcare needs within their immediate communities or society as a whole, they might be able to address gaps, thereby informing policy decisions.

Similarly, evidence-based policies in social care can support initiatives to improve the quality of care for vulnerable groups, such as older people or individuals with disabilities. Not without its risks, research-informed policies inform decisions that have impact on how health services are provided and the potential benefits to the public (Cheetham et al, 2018). This implies that policies developed based on robust research findings can address the needs of populations while promoting health equity. For example, research highlighting disparities in access to healthcare services among marginalised communities can inform policy interventions to reduce health inequalities. While research may not always lead to policy interventions or policy decision-making, research can raise awareness of challenges within health and social care services (Lancaster et al, 2020). Therefore, evidence and research-informed policy and practice are essential for health and social care services. Evidence-based practice integrates research findings, professional expertise, and client preferences to inform decision-making and service delivery (Sackett et al, 1996). By incorporating evidence from research, practitioners and students alike can ensure that interventions are grounded in the best available evidence, leading to improved outcomes for service users.

Students can consider whether or not they want their research to address disparities in healthcare services among certain groups or raise awareness of challenges within the health and social care services. This and other approaches can help students commence their research journey. Evidence-based policies in social care can support initiatives to improve the quality of care for vulnerable groups (Whitman et al, 2022). Integrating evidence from research into professional practice enables practitioners to make informed decisions, tailor interventions to individual needs, and continually improve the quality of care provided. Equally significant is the importance of this interdependency and how students conceive this understanding in the learning journey.

Student voice

As a student, it is important that you have an awareness of the significant role that research plays in health and social care practice. From my time at university, I have realised the importance of being research minded and proficient at drawing on relevant research knowledge and literature to inform my practice. This is because research gives students the opportunity to clarify processes and outcomes, it provides us with explanations, gives us an understanding of the social world, and enables students, as future professionals, to build the necessary skills and knowledge for practice.

Health and social care is a profession which has seen an unprecedented amount of change in recent years, due to austerity cuts, which has resulted in adjustments to the way services in the statutory, private, and voluntary sectors are delivered. Evidence from health and social care research influences and shapes the profession and underpins policy, and practitioners must utilise knowledge from research and other sources such as theory and law and apply this to their professional practice to provide effective services for all people who need or access health and social care services. By students showing that they understand that professional practice is supported by the best possible evidence or research, in combination with the preferences of the service users and the expertise and professional judgement of the practitioner, research bridges the gap between theoretical knowledge and practical knowledge, and the findings from research have a significant impact on the way practitioners carry out their roles. This results in research improving health and social care practice by positively impacting the way effective and appropriate services and interventions are provided for service users.

As a student, by utilising and evaluating previous research, this is likely to result in you being a more effective and competent practitioner as you will have the knowledge that will inform your professional judgements and decisions with a view to addressing service users' needs. The hierarchy of evidence provides a useful tool to help determine the best research evidence and suggests that some forms of research may be stronger and more reliable than others. The strongest evidence in health and social care interventions will come from randomised control trials, systematic reviews, and meta-analyses because they are the most valid and reliable sources, and they can collect data from large numbers of trials and other studies. As a student, utilising your library database and academic websites are the most reliable sources of finding peer reviewed research.

By acquiring knowledge about research, I feel I now have the necessary skills to put EBP into practice as I am now able to select the best possible research evidence available. I am able to do this through my knowledge of how to conduct successful literature searches. Furthermore, I now have the skills to use research knowledge to support effective decision-making when on placement in health and social care settings.

Conclusion

Research is very important in health and social care. This leads to better care for people who require assistance. This knowledge enables healthcare staff to better understand diseases, determine which therapies work best, and ultimately improve patient care. However, using research in everyday situations might prove difficult. There is a lot of information to process, and it can be difficult to adapt sophisticated research findings to real-world circumstances. Social healthcare professionals, for example, must weigh research findings against their own professional judgement, the current situation they are dealing with, as well as the wishes of their clients. The Covid-19 pandemic further demonstrated how important research is. Quick research on the virus supported public health decisions and treatment procedures, demonstrating how science may directly save lives and safeguard the public good. Practitioners are therefore required to continuously learn and reflect on their job. Reflective practice entails carefully considering their actions and decisions and conducting study to better their understanding and skills. This constant learning helps them provide better care.

Furthermore, students may apply Thompson's PCS model to identify, understand, and critique evidence from research. As explained in this chapter, students can collaborate with service users and commence their research journey by investigating disparities among other challenges that can inform policy. By incorporating evidence from research, practitioners and students alike can ensure that interventions are grounded in the best available evidence, leading to improved outcomes for service users.

In conclusion, research is essential in health and social care. It provides the necessary evidence to enhance practice, change policy, and assure high-quality care, all motivations for students to engage in research. Despite the difficulty of interpreting complicated information and barriers through policy limitations, research enables professionals to provide better care. The commitment to using research and evidence-based practice ultimately improves results for everyone who uses health and social care services.

Reflective questions

1. How do we integrate research into everyday practice, making it meaningful for people who require support?
2. To what extent can challenges associated with robust research frustrate research-informed practice and policy in health and social care?
3. How will you utilise research, theory, policy, and literature to inform and enhance your knowledge and practice?

References

Belcher, WL (2019) *Writing Your Journal Article in Twelve Weeks*. 2nd Edn. London: University of Chicago Press.

Byrne, M (2012) *How to Conduct Research for Service Improvement – A Guidebook for Health and Social Care Professionals*. HSCP Education and Development Advisory Group Research Sub-Group.

Cass, H (2024) *Independent Review of Gender Identity Services for Children and Young People*. Available at: https://cass.independent-review.uk/ (accessed 26 April 2024).

Centres for Disease Control and Prevention. (2020) *COVID-19: How to Protect Yourself and Others*. Available at: www.cdc.gov/coronavirus/2019-ncov/prevent-getting-sick/prevention.html (accessed 22 March 2024).

Cheetham, M Wiseman, A Khazaeli, B Gibson, E Gray, P Van der Graaf, P and Rushmer, R (2018) Embedded research: a promising way to create evidence-informed impact in public health? *Journal of Public Health*, 40: i64–i70.

D'Cruz, H and Jones, M (2014) *Social Work Research in Practice*. 2nd Edn. London: SAGE Publications Ltd.

Department for Science, Innovation and Technology (2021) *Independent Review of Research Bureaucracy: Final Report*. Available at: https://assets.publishing.service.gov.uk/media/62e234da8fa8f5033275fc32/independent-review-research-bureaucracy-final-report.pdf (accessed 10 September 2024).

Disability Discrimination Act 1995, c50

Equality Act (2010), c15

Gabbay, J Le May, A Pope, C Brangan, E Cameron, A Klein, JH and Wye, L (2020) Uncovering the processes of knowledge transformation: the example of local evidence-informed policy-making in United Kingdom healthcare. *Health Research Policy and Systems*, 18: 1–15.

Garrett, PM (2023) Social work and the 'social doctor': Bowlby, social reproduction and 'common sense'. *The British Journal of Social Work*, 53(1): 587–603.

Heaslip, V and Lindsay, B (2019) *Research and Evidence-Based Practice: For Nursing, Health and Social Care Students*. 1st Edn. Banbury: Lantern Publishing Limited.

Holmes, EA O'Connor, RC Perry, VH Tracey, I Wessely, S Arseneault, L and Bullmore, E (2020) Multidisciplinary research priorities for the COVID-19 pandemic: a call for action for mental health science. *The Lancet Psychiatry*, 7(6): 547–560.

Hulatt, I and Lowes, L (2005) *Involving Service Users in Health and Social Care Research*. London: Routledge.

Lancaster, K Rhodes, T and Rosengarten, M (2020) Making evidence and policy in public health emergencies: lessons from COVID-19 for adaptive evidence-making and intervention. *Evidence & Policy*, 16(3): 477–490.

Lawson, HA et al (2015) *Participatory Action Research*. 1st Edn. Oxford: Oxford University Press.

Marmot, M Allen, J Goldblatt, P Herd, E and Morrison, J (2020) *Build Back Fairer: The COVID-19 Marmot Review*. Available at: www.health.org.uk/publications/build-back-fairer-the-covid-19-marmot-review (accessed 22 March 2024).

Moule, P (2015) *Making Sense of Research in Nursing, Health and Social Care*. 5th Edn. London: SAGE Publications Ltd.

Nyström, ME Karltun, J Keller, C and Andersson Gäre, B (2018) Collaborative and partnership research for improvement of health and social services: researcher's experiences from 20 projects. *Health Research Policy and Systems*, 16: 1–17.

Perry, S (2023) 'Tory minister defends deputy chair Lee Anderson who wants to fight next election on 'trans debate''. *The Pink News*. 10 March. Available at: www.thepinknews.com/2023/03/10/sarah-dines-lee-anderson-trans-debate/ (accessed 21 June 2024).

Powell, T Baker, C and Foster, D (2024) *Capacity Pressures in Health and Social Care in England*. Available at: https://commonslibrary.parliament.uk/capacity-pressures-in-health-and-social-care-in-england/ (accessed 10 September 2024).

Public Health England (2015) *Preventing Suicide Among Trans Young People A Toolkit for Nurses*. Available at: www.gov.uk/government/publications/preventing-suicide-lesbian-gay-and-bisexual-young-people (accessed 21 June 2024).

Rajan, S Comas-Herrera, A and Mckee, M (2020) Did the UK government really throw a protective ring around care homes in the COVID-19 pandemic? *Journal of Long-Term Care*, 185–195.

Rubin, O Errett, NA Upshur, R and Baekkeskov, E (2021) The challenges facing evidence-based decision making in the initial response to COVID-19. *Scandinavian Journal of Public Health*, 49(7): 790–796.

Sackett, DL Rosenberg, WM Gray, JA Haynes, RB and Richardson, WS (1996) Evidence-based medicine: what it is and what it isn't. *BMJ: British Medical Journal*, 312(7023): 71.

Shakespeare, T (2006) *Disability Rights and Wrongs*. Oxon: Routledge.

Smith, B Williams, O Bone, L and the Moving Social Work Co-production Collective (2023) Co-production: a resource to guide co-producing research in the sport, exercise, and health sciences. *Qualitative Research in Sport, Exercise and Health*, 15(2): 159–187.

Stepney, P and Thompson, N (2021) Isn't it time to start "theorising practice" rather than trying to "apply theory to practice"? Reconsidering our approach to the relationship between theory and practice. *Practice (Birmingham, England)*, 33(2): 149–163.

Strehlenert, H Richter-Sundberg, L Nyström, ME and Hasson, H (2015) Evidence-informed policy formulation and implementation: a comparative case study of two national policies for improving health and social care in Sweden. *Implementation Science*, 10: 1–10.

Thompson, N (2020) *Anti-Discriminatory Practice*. 7th Edn. London: Bloomsbury Publishing Plc.

Webb, SA (2001) Some considerations on the validity of evidence-based practice in social work. *The British Journal of Social Work*, 31(1): 57–79.

Whitman, A De Lew, N Chappel, A Aysola, V Zuckerman, R and Sommers, BD (2022) Addressing social determinants of health: examples of successful evidence-based strategies and current federal efforts. *Off Health Policy*, 1: 1–30.

World Health Organization (2020) *COVID-19 Vaccines*. Available at: www.who.int/emergencies/diseases/novel-coronavirus-2019/covid-19-vaccines (accessed 22 March 2024).

CHAPTER 4

Ethical considerations in health and social care research

Jessica Eve Jackson, Lesley Deacon, Tess King and Ola Tony-Obot

Introduction

As practitioners we are expected to act ethically, following principles of integrity and transparency and making decisions that prioritise service-users' well-being and rights. In research, ethics is vital to fostering trust, reliability, and responsible practice in pursuing knowledge. Clark et al (2021) highlight that ethical research frameworks change and develop as new areas of knowledge emerge. Something considered ethical in the past may not be today, and knowledge production changes must lead us to reconsider how we engage ethically. For example, increased online activity means we must consider ethics of personal data, despite that data being openly available in the public domain. Ethical thinking is integral to the research process and should not be ignored but explored.

Chapter concepts

This chapter explores how we recognise and respond to ethical research dilemmas using practical approaches, across the following five areas:

- Moral thinking and the origins of research ethics governance.
- The use of self to recognise ethical practices.
- Conflicts of ethics as an early-career practitioner-researcher.
- Embedding ethics at every step.
- Responding to ethical considerations.

Throughout we use the term practitioner-researcher to demonstrate the positionality of those of us who are within a field of practice (such as nursing or social work) while also conducting research in practice settings (Flynn and McDermott, 2016; Deacon, 2023).

DOI: 10.4324/9781041056782-6

Moral thinking and the origins of research ethics governance

Ethics in research is not a static concept, but one that raises issues for consideration and debate. According to Banks (2012), there are different ethical concepts: *meta*, *normative*, and *descriptive*. *Meta* concerns how we determine what is right; *normative* concerns guiding principles that should be followed in any situation; *descriptive* concerns people's moral opinions and how they act on them (Deacon, 2017). As individuals, we all have moral principles that guide our actions (Grix, 2019), and may also be guided by professional ethics; for example, the Social Work England professional ethical principle, stipulating respect and dignity when interacting with service-users, or the Nursing and Midwifery Council's Code of Professional Practice, whose purpose is to guide our conduct as practitioners. Additionally, we have research ethics governance guided by our organisations, such as Higher Education Institutions and/or the NHS. These emerged from codes and declarations following serious concerns around unethical medical research: the Nuremberg Code (1949) established ten key moral, ethical, and legal principles for human research (Flynn and McDermott, 2016); following this, the Declaration of Helsinki (1964), from the World Medical Association, set international standards. Key principles include respect for research participants and their potential vulnerability.

Although we have research governance to guide ethical thinking, debates concerning ethical research decisions are still widespread. Clark et al (2021) highlight different standpoints in ethical decisions: from a universalistic position, where ethical rules should be followed no matter what (deontology), to a flexible approach suggesting the ends justify the means (utilitarianism/consequentialism). This highlights that, despite ethical research guidelines, the concept of ethics remains contested and complex, and due diligence is needed to ensure research is ethical.

The use of self to recognise ethical practices

Research in professional settings has additional ethical considerations. The importance of reflecting on our positionality uses the self to recognise ethical practice, and identifying ethical conflicts when they arise is essential. For ethical research, we must embed ethical decision-making throughout designing, conducting, analysing, and reporting, rather than only when applying for ethical approval.

As practitioner-researchers in specialist practice, we can potentially contribute to knowledge and advancements in our fields, and positively impact real-world issues. We must consider these potential outcomes alongside possible impacts on individual research participants. Once ethical approval is obtained from organisations/institutions, we may think we are ideally positioned to collect workplace data. However, as practitioner-researchers, we may be working among the providers of our research data: patients, service-users, and colleagues. This necessitates ethical reflection early in the process of research development.

Ethical consideration should be given to our potential privileged access to sensitive data, observations, and experiences (Saidin, 2017) (see Chapters 4 and 5). In these circumstances we must consider consequences of data access and use it responsibly. We must also consider our relationships with research participants. As practitioners we may regularly engage with patients or service-users, but as researchers we need to consider how participants may perceive research and receive our engagement (Jackson et al, 2024) (see Chapter 5). A Health Visitor researching parents' experiences of their service may be tempted to consult people they expect to be willing to share experiences, but this introduces potential bias, as only certain views are sought, and marginalised voices may go unheard. This does not suggest *intentional* bias, but as practitioner-researchers engaged in active practice we must ensure we always explore our assumptions and reflect on the following core ethical principles (Varkey, 2021):

- *Autonomy*: respecting an individual's right to make decisions and choices.
- *Beneficence*: acting in the best interest of others, promoting good and preventing harm.
- *Nonmaleficence*: avoiding actions that cause harm or injury to others.
- *Justice*: ensuring fair and equitable treatment and distribution of resources.
- *Confidentiality*: protecting private information, ensuring it is shared only with appropriate parties.

Practitioner-researchers additionally experience conflicts due to our position as insiders/outsiders. We can be *insiders* if research is conducted within our organisation/profession, but considered *outsiders* if we have left the profession, e.g. into academia. This conflict is inextricably linked to our positioning within our research; practitioner-researchers are trained within a specific value base but must separate this from our position within research.

Bassot (2020) recommends *reflexivity* to explore our values and beliefs and their influence on our actions, using self-awareness and critical thinking to ensure ethical decision-making. Reflexivity is a sociological concept encouraging us to consider our position in society and how that influences our views in our practice and decision-making (Bourdieu and Wacquant, 1992). Whilst reflection is a static consideration of our actions, *reflexivity* is ongoing and fluid, exploring in-depth our values and integrity, and how they impact on participants, building trust and credibility into our research. Bassot (2020) suggests this influences our thoughts and acknowledges our different perceptions in our roles as researchers and as practitioners.

Reflective question

How can our dual responsibilities as practitioners and researchers be balanced to ensure *autonomy, beneficence, nonmaleficence, justice,* and *confidentiality* of participants are prioritised while maintaining integrity and ethical standards of research?

Conflicts of ethics as an early-career practitioner-researcher

A core ethical research decision-making principle is *nonmaleficence* – avoidance of harm to participants/researchers (Clark et al, 2021). However, early-career practitioner-researchers face challenges navigating time-consuming research processes or balancing demands of a university programme with professional duties. Additionally, Deacon (2023) highlights that practitioner-researchers have the skills to conduct research but lack confidence naming what they do as research. This can deter engagement in research, presenting identity conflict for practitioner-researchers who have less confidence in their decision-making.

Health and social care practitioners engage in reflection during professional training, e.g. Schön's (1984) *reflective practitioner*. Practitioners also develop reflection skills promoting ongoing learning and good practice, considering what knowledge and values this brings to practice, and how this impacts interactions and decisions (Comer, 2016). One outcome of reflective practice is self-awareness of bias and consideration of actions taken, thereby enhancing ethical awareness within research. This ensures research is ethical, identifying the challenges that may arise, developing research questions, alternative perspectives on topics, power dynamics between researcher and participants, potential impacts on participants and how to minimise these.

Reflective question

You are embarking on a new research project as a practitioner in an area of practice where you have expertise. What existing knowledge and experiences might help you consider ethical issues as you approach this new practitioner-researcher role?

Embedding ethics at every step

Different professionals may require different processes for ethical approvals. However, all health and social care researchers must obtain correct approvals from *all* organisations involved before commencing (De Poli and Oyebode, 2023). Ethics committees assess how key principles are addressed in our planned process, ensuring the rights, welfare, and dignity of all participants are respected and protected. Explicit ethics criteria might include how research involves people, obtains consent, maintains confidentiality, provides a withdrawal procedure, and ensures an appropriate methodological approach (Post and Blustein, 2021).

As researchers, we might disagree with ethics committee requests/decisions, especially if we feel the committee is overly restrictive or misunderstands aspects of the study (Kohn and Shore, 2017). In such cases, we can seek clarification, revise/resubmit the proposal, or appeal the decision. However, in the event of ethics committee rejection, researchers typically revise their proposals to address concerns and learn from feedback. Rejection, while frustrating, is a common part of the learning process in academic research (Chan et al, 2021).

Involvement

Involving the public in research has developed significantly in recent years, also termed inclusive, participatory, action, or emancipatory research (Nind, 2021). It is good practice to involve the wider public in research design and delivery. The National Institute for Health and Care Research (2024) set out value-based *UK Standards for Public Involvement* in research, to support self-reflection and learning. They describe good public involvement and recommend inclusive opportunities are provided in our research, actively fostering an environment where individuals from diverse backgrounds feel welcome and empowered to participate and contribute. We do this by collaborating with interested community groups, ensuring our research is relevant, responsive, and disseminated to a wider audience. We may ask people with relevant life experience to review participant-facing research documents, ensuring communication is inclusive and accessible.

There are good examples of collaboration and co-production with historically excluded populations, e.g. Jackson et al's (2023) collaboration with transgender and non-binary parents with multidisciplinary healthcare professionals to design, deliver, analyse, and report findings of a study exploring chestfeeding and breastfeeding experiences. The team met regularly to plan research goals, and processes, and agree on data collection tools and approaches. The team was also equally involved in analysis and reporting.

Despite increasing involvement in research, more consideration is needed to proactively increase inclusivity in research and address systemic disparities for minority groups. It is crucial to consider how people are compensated for offering their time and given recognition for their contributions, avoiding exploitation (Pearce, 2021). Where research aligns with community or social causes, participants may want to contribute if they feel their involvement will have a positive societal impact. Therefore, it is important to show how involvement contributes to the greater good, especially in nonprofit or public health-related research (Jackson et al, 2024). Offering flexible, time-efficient involvement with an opportunity to be acknowledged in publications can also be an incentive.

> ### Reflective question
>
> How would you involve the wider community and service-users in designing your research study, ensuring their contributions are recognised?

Recruitment

Recruiting participants from practice can be ethically challenging because of potential power imbalances in professional relationships, leading to service-users feeling pressure to participate. Asking 'gatekeepers' (colleagues with access to potential participants or settings in which research is conducted) to recruit may also influence participants' decisions to join a study, potentially introducing bias or coercion (Guillemin et al, 2017). Although this can help reduce pressure felt by service-users in direct care, an ethical concern remains that patients might feel obliged to join because the recommendation comes from someone they trust. Anybody recruiting should clearly explain the study, and ensure potential participants understand participation is voluntary and will not affect their care. Clear, honest communication and respecting their autonomy help balance the need for research with patients' right to make their choices without coercion (Varkey, 2021).

Consent

Ensuring respondents can give 'informed consent' is essential. It is also crucial to consider how we can be confident that potential participants fully understand the study and what taking part involves (Godskesen et al, 2023). Practitioner-researchers can also consider the principle '*do no harm*' when considering the potential impact of participating, and supporting people to make an informed choice. Participants should be given time and space to understand and consider all information, and to ask any questions. However, other types of consent might be more suitable for different study designs and certain population groups.

Table 4.1 offers examples of common ways to obtain consent, their application and theoretical underpinnings, although it is not an exhaustive list.

An approach to practice-based, practitioner-led research is *Facilitated Practice-based Research* (FPR) (copyright University of Sunderland) (Deacon, 2023), a model based on principles of empowerment and universal design, to decrease practitioner-researcher anxiety and increase confidence. In each programme cohort, practitioner-researchers work together to co-construct an area of relevant practice-based research. One example

Table 4.1 Types of consent, their application and theoretical underpinnings

Consent	Application	Theoretical underpinning
Implied consent assumes the participant is aware of the situation and would voluntarily agree to terms or conditions.	Anonymous questionnaires or low-risk research design where participation is non-invasive (Stokes et al, 2019).	Principle of reasonable expectation, where participation is assumed through action (returning a completed questionnaire), thus eliminating the need for explicit consent (Moreno et al, 2013).
Verbal consent is explicit, spoken agreement to participate where individuals assert their rights through direct communication.	Informal settings, phone, or online interviews, where written consent may cause discomfort, where participants have limited literacy (Tamariz et al, 2013).	Principle of autonomy, where there is a mutual understanding that spoken consent indicates agreement, provided both parties can comprehend informed decisions in the given context (Spector, 2022).
Parental/guardian consent is a legal and ethical requirement for a parent or guardian to permit their minor to participate in a study.	Research involving minors who cannot legally consent for themselves. It is good practice to obtain *assent* from the minor, as an agreement to take part in an age-appropriate manner (Weisleder, 2020).	Principle of protection and substituted judgement where parents or guardians act in the child's best interest. It draws on the concept of diminished autonomy, recognising that children require safeguarding (White, 2020).
Proxy consent can be obtained from a legally authorised representative such as a guardian or caregiver.	Where the participant is unable to do so, such as an unconscious patient or someone with cognitive impairments (Shepherd, 2022).	Principle of beneficence, where opportunity is afforded, acknowledging substituted judgement standard, where the proxy makes decisions based on what they believe the individual would want, thereby safeguarding their interests and rights (Avant and Swetz, 2020).

explored what 'consent' looked like and how it was experienced by families, which raised these ethical issues:

- How to access potential participants without breaching Data Protection.
- How to ensure practitioner-researchers do not know the people they are interviewing.
- How to guarantee people were giving informed consent to participate.

To address these concerns, adverts were sent to families with their closing letters from the organisation. Once participants were known, practitioner-researchers were asked to confirm whether they knew the person, and if they did, they did not conduct the interview. The project lead engaged with participants over consent, ensuring it was made clear regarding their right not to participate.

Reflective question

You are recruiting for your study to explore experiences of a new intervention. A potential participant, an elderly individual with mild cognitive impairment, expresses interest in joining the study. The cognitive impairment may affect their ability to provide fully informed consent. What steps will you take to address this, to enable them to participate?

Debrief and withdrawal

Debriefing participants following involvement ensures they receive necessary follow-up information. It also fulfils the principle of informed consent, as participants are made aware of the study's true purpose, any deception used, and how their data will be handled. Deception can only be used if revealing the true purpose of a study before participation would alter behaviour, thus compromising the validity of results. For example, Bunten et al (2021) took photographs of children's primary school packed lunches, with the school's consent, before providing health promotion packed lunch resources for children to take home to their parents. They then took further photographs post-intervention and at follow-up to measure any reduction in high-sugar and high-fat products. The parents were fully debriefed following the study. However, if they had been told photographs would be taken before the study commenced it may have influenced what they would normally pack for their child for lunch during that school day.

Inadequate explanation of a study can leave participants confused or distrustful, and may cause participants to feel upset, embarrassed, or distressed when revealing full details, particularly for sensitive topics. We must address potential harm and provide necessary support/referrals. Opportunity for debrief is often a regulatory requirement, reflecting the ethical obligation to respect participants' autonomy and dignity, so clear and informative debriefing materials are essential. University ethics committees offer templates/resources to ensure debriefing covers key elements: purpose of study, potential misconceptions, and participants' rights. Additionally, a robust withdrawal procedure allows participants to exercise their right to stop involvement without consequence, ensuring they are not coerced or pressured to remain against their wishes. The withdrawal process must be clearly explained before obtaining consent.

Confidentiality, analysing, and reporting

Confidentiality in research means protecting participants' identities/data from unauthorised access or disclosure, often through encryption or secure storage. Deontological ethics, particularly Kantian ethics, supports confidentiality by upholding the moral duty to respect individuals' intrinsic right to privacy, irrespective of consequences (Varden, 2020). The duty to maintain confidentiality aligns with treating participants as individuals with rights to dignity and respect, not merely tools for research goals. This ethical responsibility is critical to building trust and ensuring participants feel secure.

Anonymity goes further by ensuring no identifying information about participants is collected or retained, completely shielding their identities from the researcher. Anonymity is part of a social contract between researcher and participant, where participants agree to provide data under implicit understanding that their identities will be protected. Trust in research is built on ethical reciprocity (Su et al, 2021). However, it may not be possible for practitioner-researchers to recruit participants anonymously. Therefore, maintaining confidentiality of identifiable, sensitive, personal, or medical information when reporting results is crucial, and requires adherence to organisation policy and law (UK Legislation, 2018). We can maintain confidentiality of participants by assigning unique identification codes or pseudonyms to replace identifiable information, ensuring participants' identities are not directly linked to data. We can also report findings in aggregate form, preventing identification of any individual participant in published results.

Poor methodological analysis raises several ethical concerns. It could waste resources, cause misleading or unreproducible findings, or violate trust, increasing risk of harm to participants. Utilitarianism theorises that moral rightness of actions is determined by consequences (Mill, 2016); inefficient, wasteful research contradicts the principle of maximising benefits while minimising harm to participants and society. Addressing these ethical concerns requires researchers to prioritise methodological rigour, through peer review, ethics committee feedback, mentors/supervisors, or workshops/seminars.

Practitioner research occurs in professional settings often with dominant ideologies and political climates and can be seen as challenging the status quo. For ethical reporting, we must articulate a clear vision to engage leaders through transparent communication and involvement in decision-making, perhaps through presenting findings through workshops/seminars. It is also important to share findings with the population they impact. The Public Understanding of Science (PUS) movement advocates for enhancing public knowledge and appreciation of science (Lewis et al, 2023) and highlights the need for researchers to communicate findings in accessible ways, bridging the gap between academia and the public, fostering trust and understanding. Traditional dissemination of findings, e.g. publication in academic journals or presenting at conferences, often excludes the people the research is for/about, so it is important to consider alternative ways to share findings, such as multimedia films or infographics.

Reflective question

What would you do if members of your organisation were not happy with your research findings?

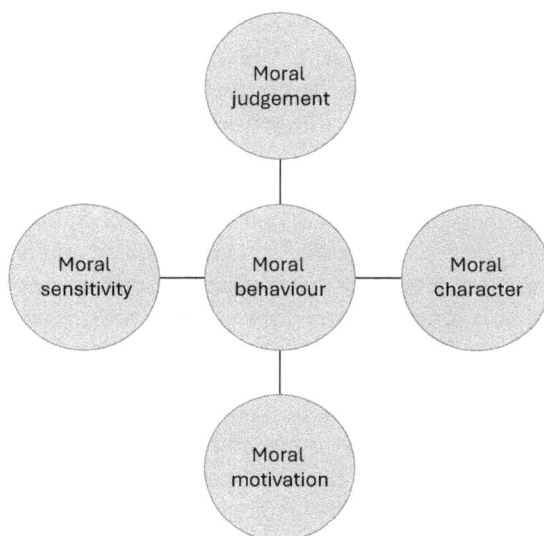

Figure 4.1 Rest's Four-Component Model of Moral Behaviour

Responding to ethical considerations

When practitioner-researchers encounter unexpected ethical dilemmas, we should follow a structured process to ensure our response is thoughtful, informed, and aligned with ethical standards. Imagine you are conducting a study, and data from one participant reveals a serious condition unrelated to your investigation. Disclosing this could benefit the participant but breaches confidentiality. You may decide to disclose the information, prioritising the participant's well-being, but this would need careful consideration and appropriate justification.

- First consider our ethical guidelines on participant confidentiality and disclosure.
- Also consider ethical principles such as beneficence (potential benefit) and confidentiality.
- Also discuss the dilemma and planned action with our supervisor.

After these steps, if you decide to inform the participant, it should be confidentially and sensitively, ensuring they understand the context and implications. In this circumstance, you should review the process and outcome and document the experience for future reference. Rest's Four-Component Model of Moral Behaviour (Vozzola, 2016) outlines four components necessary for ethical decision-making (see Figure 4.1). Using this model to structure approaches to ethical dilemmas as practitioner-researchers helps ensure they are handled responsibly, balancing principles with practical considerations.

Student voices

I find it helpful to stay in tune with social work ethical principles of upholding dignity and respect when interacting with participants/service-users, as stipulated in the ethical guidelines. However, I struggled to stay in my role as researcher and not allow my views to influence participants, since we somehow share similar experiences of the research.

However, being a reflexive practitioner-researcher has enhanced my understanding of research ethics, assisting me in navigating the dilemma and allowing me to adhere to the moral principle of respecting participants' views throughout the research. Having a clear understanding of ethics relating to openness and respect, as well as being reflective, I found it useful to prevent the likelihood of infringing on participants' values and integrity. I should emphasise always reflecting at every step of the research as similarly done within good practice standards to help navigate ethical dilemmas.

I drew on previous experience to consider whether participants could give informed consent, maintaining confidentiality, and balancing my interest in completing the research with asking someone to share their experiences, recognising the potential impact of this. It is important to consider the similarities and differences between my practice role and research. Perspectives and values are similar, based on personal and professional experiences and influences, but one key difference in the roles is connected to power. Potentially, there could be differences in the power my professional role holds, compared to that of a researcher, particularly depending on the nature of my practice (child protection, mental health). Some ethical concerns appear more straightforward to me: promoting choice, informed consent, and opportunities to withdraw. Others are more challenging: promoting the principle of doing no harm and considering/minimising potential impact for participants. The focus on reflexivity supported me in reflecting on how my approach, values, perspectives, and biases could influence the research process.

Conclusion

This chapter has explored key principles specifically for practitioner-researchers to enable reflection on, recognition of, and response to ethical dilemmas related to conducting research in a practice setting. It has highlighted key practical approaches used throughout the research process with illustrative examples.

As demonstrated, practitioner-researchers have unique opportunities to contribute to practice advancements and facilitate positive outcomes for our population's health and social care. However, reflecting on the positionality between the two potentially conflicting professional roles of practitioner and researcher is crucial in the responsible pursuit of knowledge. As early-career practitioner-researchers, we may also face challenges balancing the demands of our roles. However, as trained practitioners, we can use our existing reflective skills to underpin ethical decision-making.

The most important theme within this chapter is the understanding that ethics needs to be considered and embedded at every step of the research process. It is not just something to address when applying for ethical approval. It is beyond the scope of this chapter to explore every ethical encounter possible during research. We are likely to encounter unexpected ethical dilemmas, and to address these we must follow a structured process, adhering to ethical guidelines and principles, reflecting and discussing these with our supervisors to consider appropriate responses.

References

Avant, LC and Swetz, KM (2020) Revisiting beneficence: what is a 'benefit', and by what criteria? *The American Journal of Bioethics*, 20(3): 75–77.

Banks, S (2012) *Ethics and Values in Social Work*. London: Palgrave-MacmIllan.

Bassot, B (2020) *The Reflective Journal*. 3rd Edn. London: Bloomsbury.

Bourdieu, P and Wacquant, L (1992) *An Invitation to Reflexive Sociology*. Cambridge: Blackwell.

Bunten, A Porter, L Burgess-Allen, J Howell-Jones, R Jackson, J Ward, D Staples, V Staples, P Rowthorn, H Saei, A and Van Schaik, P (2021) Using behavioural insights to reduce sugar in primary school children's packed lunches in Derby: a cluster randomised controlled trial. *Appetite*, 157: 104987.

Chan, H Mazzucchelli, TG and Rees, CS (2021) The battle-hardened academic: an exploration of the resilience of university academics in the face of ongoing criticism and rejection of their research. *Higher Education Research & Development*, 40(3): 446–460.

Clark, T Foster, L Sloan, L and Brymna, A (2021) *Bryman's Social Research Methods*. 6th Edn. Oxford: Oxford University Press.

Comer, M (2016) Rethinking reflection-in-action: what did Schön really mean? *Nurse education today*, 36: 4–6.

De Poli, C and Oyebode, J (2023) Research ethics and collaborative research in health and social care: analysis of UK research ethics policies, scoping review of the literature, and focus group study. *Plos one*, 18(12): e0296223.

Deacon, L (2017) Ethical and moral philosophies. In: Deacon, L and Macdonald, SJ (eds) *Social Work Theories and Practice*. London: Sage Publications, pp 113–114.

Deacon, L (2023) Facilitated practice-based research: a model of empowerment to reduce research anxiety in social work practitioners and reframe cultural capital. *European Journal of Social Work Research*, 1(1): 102–117.

Flynn, C and McDermott, F (2016) *Doing Research in Social Work and Social Care: The journey from student to practitioner researcher*. London: SAGE Publications.

Godskesen, T, Björk, J and Juth, N (2023) Challenges regarding informed consent in recruitment to clinical research: a qualitative study of clinical research nurses' experiences. *Trials*, 24(1): 801.

Guillemin, M McDougall, R Martin, D Hallowell, N Brookes, A and Gillam, L (2017) Primary care physicians' views about gatekeeping in clinical research recruitment: a qualitative study. *AJOB Empirical Bioethics*, 8(2): 99–105.

Grix, J (2019) *The Foundations of Research*. 3rd Edn. London: Red Globe Press.

Jackson, JE Wild, R Hallam, J Graves, R Woodstein, BJ and Stothard, P (2023) Exploring the healthcare experiences and support needs of chestfeeding or breastfeeding for trans and non-binary parents based in the United Kingdom. *International Journal of Transgender Health*, 25(4): 738–750 https://doi.org/10.1080/26895269.2023.2265371.

Jackson, JE Moreton, J Barnett, N and Hurst, M (2024) Understanding how nurses can effectively utilise social media for increasing public involvement, recruitment and impact dissemination of clinical research trials. *Journal of Research in Nursing*, 29(4–5): 321–331.https://doi.org/10.1177/17449871241246963.

Kohn, T and Shore, C (2017) The ethics of university ethics committees, risk management and the research imagination. In: Wright, S and Shore, C (eds) *Death of the Public University*. Oxford and New York: Berghahn Books, pp 229–249.

Lewis, J Bartlett, A Riesch, H and Stephens, N (2023) Why we need a public understanding of social science. *Public Understanding of Science*, 32(5): 658–672.

Mill, JS (2016) Utilitarianism. In: Cahn, SM (ed) *Seven Masterpieces of Philosophy*. London: Routledge, pp 329–375.

Moreno, MA Goniu, N Moreno, PS and Diekema, D (2013) Ethics of social media research: common concerns and practical considerations. *Cyberpsychology, Behavior, and Social Networking*, 16(9): 708–713.

National Institute for Health and Care Research (2024) *UK Standards for Public Involvement*. Available at: https://sites.google.com/nihr.ac.uk/pi-standards/home (accessed 13 March 2024).

Nind, M (2021) *Inclusive Research*. London: Bloomsbury.

Pearce, C (2021) The complexities of developing equal relationships in patient and public involvement in health research. *Social Theory & Health*, 19: 362–379.

Post, LF and Blustein, J (2021) *Handbook for Health Care Ethics Committees*. Baltimore: JHU Press.

Saidin, K (2017) Insider researchers: challenges and opportunities. *Proceedings of the ICECRS*, 1(1): 849–854. doi:10.21070/picecrs.v1i1.563.

Schön, DA (1984) *The Reflective Practitioner: How Professionals Think in Action*. New York: Basic Books.

Shepherd, V (2022) (Re)conceptualising 'good' proxy decision-making for research: the implications for proxy consent decision quality. *BMC Medical Ethics*, 23(1): 75.

Spector, H (2022) Autonomy and rights. In: Colburn, B (ed) *The Routledge Handbook of Autonomy*. London: Routledge, pp 313–323.

Stokes, Y Vandyk, A Squires, J Jacob, JD and Gifford, W (2019) Using Facebook and LinkedIn to recruit nurses for an online survey. *Western Journal of Nursing Research*, 41(1): 96–110.

Su, X Lin, W Wu, J Zheng, Q Chen, X and Jiang, X (2021) Ethical leadership and knowledge sharing: the effects of positive reciprocity and moral efficacy. *Sage Open*, 11(2): 21582440211021823.

Tamariz, L Palacio, A Robert, M and Marcus, EN (2013) Improving the informed consent process for research subjects with low literacy: a systematic review. *Journal of General Internal Medicine*, 28: 121–126.

UK Legislation (2018) *General Data Protection Regulation (GDPR)*. Available at: www.legislation.gov.uk/ukpga/2018/12/contents/enacted (accessed 14 June 2024).

Varden, H (2020) Kantian care. In: Bhandary, A and Baehr, AR (eds) *Caring for Liberalism*. London: Routledge, pp 50–74.

Varkey, B (2021) Principles of clinical ethics and their application to practice. *Medical Principles and Practice*, 30(1): 17–28.

Vozzola, EC (2016) The case for the four component model vs. moral foundations theory: a perspective from moral psychology. *Mercer L. Rev.*, 68: 633.

Weisleder, P (2020) Helping them decide: a scoping review of interventions used to help minors understand the concept and process of assent. *Frontiers in Pediatrics*, 8: 25.

White, MG (2020) Why human subjects research protection is important. *Ochsner Journal*, 20(1): 16–33.

CHAPTER 5

Managing the relationship

Chantelle Taylor and Hazel Spence

Introduction

Using a case study of an online parenting support group for parents of SEND (Special Education Needs and Disabilities) children, this chapter explores how a researcher's identity affects their relationship with the research, the readers, the participants, and the ivory tower of academia. Traditionally it was deemed necessary to write yourself out of research to appear objective, scientific, and *good*. This chapter will illustrate that writing yourself into your research is beneficial for wider society, the researcher, the reader, the research participants, and the overall institution of academia.

Chapter concepts
- Managing the relationship with your research
- Managing the relationship with your readers
- Managing the relationship with your participants
- Managing the relationship with the ivory tower

Reflective questions

When reading this chapter, reflect on how your identity has impacted on your own research. Think about why you chose to study your topic. Has your own lived experience influenced how and what you are researching?

DOI: 10.4324/9781041056782-7

Case study

A researcher is studying how parents of children with SEND use social media for support. Using digital ethnography, the researcher observes a private Facebook group for parents of SEND children. The researcher thematically analyses the anonymous posts written on the group wall, looking for shared codes and themes. Some of the anonymous posts talk about extremely sensitive information such as mental health and suicide, and domestic abuse and violence. Some of the parents on the group share incredibly detailed, confidential information about their children.

The researcher is a parent of SEND children. The researcher was already a member of the closed Facebook group prior to the start of their research. The researcher has both posted anonymously on the group wall asking for support and advice and commented on other people's posts offering the same. The researcher has shared information to the group about their own vulnerable children.

Using autoethnography the researcher has also shared their own experiences of using social media for SEND support within the research project. The researcher has not disclosed to the group their identity as a researcher (other than to the group founder when asking for consent to study the group). The researcher continues to use the closed Facebook group for their own personal support after their research project has concluded.

Researcher identity

How does the researcher's identity affect the research process?

Positionality refers to the standpoint of the researcher regarding the research project, including the topic and context of the study and the participants involved (Fenge et al, 2019). A researcher's positionality is influenced by their worldview, philosophical assumptions, and background, all of which are shaped by the researcher's class, gender, race, sexuality, religion, and nationality (Folkes, 2023).

Whether consciously or unconsciously, the researcher's life experiences, due to the aforementioned characteristics, will influence the research process from the initial formulation of the research aims and questions, right through to their findings and data analysis (Morrow and Kettle, 2024). Your positionality not only affects the research questions and data findings, but it also affects every single stage of the research process, including your theoretical underpinnings and whether, for example, you use Foucault's theory of power, Marx's class theory, or Black feminist intersectionality theory (Cuevas-Parra, 2023).

Your positionality also encompasses the social, political, and cultural context in which we write (Bukamal, 2022). For example, when researching police brutality, a Black African American male researcher is going to have different lived experience and thus different positionality than a white female researcher. And both will have a differing positionality from a Black female researcher. Whether the research is conducted before or after the world watched George Floyd call out for his 'mama', or whether the research is conducted in America or England, the circumstances that surround the researcher all influence the research project.

In the case study the researcher does not have to disclose to the readers that they themselves are a SEND parent or that they are an active participant within the group that they are studying. In fact, some might say that the mere mention of the subjective side of the researcher might bias the research. However, through the disclosure of the researcher's positionality, feminists argue research is enhanced by giving the audience the opportunity to make their own minds up about the research results now they have the background information (Frances, 2023; Cooper and Rogers, 2015).

You have probably heard the words 'you must be reflexive' within the academic literature. Reflexivity requires us as researchers to have a critical awareness of how our subjective experiences, cultural background, and social positions impact our research design, data collection, and analysis (Karcher et al, 2024). It involves researchers clearly disclosing their positionality including their personal beliefs and values (Folkes, 2023). This helps researchers communicate how these factors influence their research ensuring transparency in the findings. Keeping a reflexive journal throughout the research process helps document personal biases, emotions, and reflections (Deblasio, 2022).

The inclusion of reflexive journalling into our research write ups allows for our personal experiences and subjective viewpoints to be visible throughout our research, and importantly to our research audience. In the case study the researcher claimed that within their research write up they shared their own autoethnographic experiences of using social media for SEND support. The regular sharing of first-person perspectives, including thoughts, feelings, and experiences throughout the research process, acknowledges the researcher's central role and allows for a critical reflection and an enhanced self-awareness of how we as researchers impact our research.

By consistently documenting any changes in thinking or methodology that may occur due to our positionality, particularly over long projects, we provide our readers with an audit trail that again enhances our transparency and rigour in the research process.

Historically seeing the researcher within their work was frowned upon; it went against the scientific grain that positivists had us believe we must follow to be good researchers (Ettorre, 2017).

The narrative turn and the rise of feminist methodologies has left us all scrambling to be more reflexive, yet the challenge is accepting this and doing this effectively. As Folkes (2023, p 1304) writes, reflexivity is more than just a 'shopping list' of descriptions. Reflexivity involves more than just listing our characteristics as researchers and how they are dis/like that of our participants. Reflexivity is about critically engaging (Folkes, 2023). Reflexivity is making a case to continuously challenge your research choices, your methodological decisions, your analysis, and discussion which are all based on your positionality (Morrow and Kettle, 2024). As the literature informs us, we as researchers must be continuously self-critical, self-analytical, and reflective. As such, identifying and acknowledging our own bias is not enough, we need to reflect on them and challenge them.

Writing to the reader

How can writing directly to your readers increase the integrity of your research?

Unlike positivist research which aims to minimise bias to appear objective, subjective feminist research recognises that there is always bias, and instead of trying to eradicate something that cannot be eliminated within the social world, feminists acknowledge and address such bias. Recognising bias within feminist research involves being reflexive, transparent, ethical, and recognising intersectionality and considering how intersecting identities impact both the research process and the findings. The use of reflexivity and transparency throughout your research can enhance the rigour and authenticity of your work. By being open and honest about each phase of your research and how you, and your life experiences, have influenced your work allows you to build a rapport with your readers that can challenge traditional academic boundaries. By fostering a dialogic relationship and encouraging readers to critically engage with the text, researchers break the fourth wall, creating a more interactive and engaging narrative whereby readers become directly involved within the research process (Armstrong, 2008). Aligning with feminist methodologies that emphasise reflexive, transparent knowledge that invites readers to question power dynamics and contribute to the discourse, research becomes more accessible, relatable, and promotes a deeper understanding of feminist issues.

Acknowledging our positionality and disclosing it to the reader allows us to build a relationship with our audience, it allows for reflexivity, transparency, and credibility (Folkes, 2023). As such, the reader becomes an active part of the research (Weatherall, 2023), they gain the knowledge and power to assess the impact of the researcher on the study, thus improving the quality of the research. In the case study, you can imagine there is a clear connection between being a SEND parent looking for support and researching how SEND parents access support online. Where positionality comes in is when you as a researcher make this clear to your readers.

Breaking the fourth wall challenges traditional notions of objectivity and researcher neutrality (Boivin and CohenMiller, 2018). By acknowledging the researcher's presence and perspectives, breaking the fourth wall aligns with feminist goals of empowerment.

We are not neutral, nor should we strive to be, instead we must account for the influence our active being has on our research, confronting both our personal assumptions and our ontological and epistemological ones too (Ettorre, 2017).

Ontology refers to the study of the nature of being existence and reality. Ontology seeks to understand the fundamental components that make up the social world (institutions, norms, relationships) and how these are constructed, maintained, and transformed over time (Stanley and Wise, 2002). As such, feminist ontology examines the nature of being through a feminist lens, focusing on how gender shapes our understanding of reality. Epistemology refers to the study of knowledge, focusing on how we know what we know. It explores the nature, origin, and limits of human knowledge, addressing questions about belief, truth, and justification (Stanley and Wise, 2002). Epistemology examines how knowledge is acquired and validated. Accordingly, feminist epistemology challenges the notion of objective knowledge, arguing that all knowledge is socially situated and influenced by the knower's context, including gender, race, and class. Feminist epistemology emphasises the importance of incorporating the perspectives of women and other marginalised groups, which are often excluded from traditional research. Feminist epistemology stresses understanding knowledge within its social and historical context, highlighting how power dynamics shape what is considered valid knowledge. Who we are as people and as researchers influences our methodological choices and therefore rather than trying to ignore this, we must lean into it and see ourselves as positive influences on our work; after all, researchers are not detached observers. They bring their own experiences, biases, and perspectives to the research process and this embodiment influences how they formulate questions, interpret data, and engage with participants and readers.

Positionality is outlining how you as a researcher, as a real person with lived experience, interact with the data differently to that of a researcher with differing personal characteristics, worldviews, and subjective experiences. Reflexivity is critically asking yourself, at each stage, how your own position influences each research and methodological decision; we all have bias. When we become researchers, we do not stop being people. We are not rocks. We are individuals with feelings, thoughts, and emotions. Instead of claiming that we can be objective and removed from personal bias, value judgement and subjective influence, let us make clear to our readers, our subjectivities, and the influences that they have. Let us give the readers the knowledge and the power to make their own decisions on the impact and candour of our research. What motivates us is our experiences and what motivates our research is a strive to improve the lives of those like us (Morrow and Kettle, 2024). As such, to achieve these goals we often must study those with whom we closely align.

The researcher's relationship
What happens when the researcher is part of the researched?

In the case study, although conducted behind closed screens and without the other members of the group being aware, the researcher as a SEND parent can still be classed as an insider. In this circumstance the researcher is a complete member researcher – this is often an observational (covert/overt, participatory/non-participatory) methodology where the researcher is fully immersed within the group in which they are studying (McNarry et al, 2024).

A well-known and often-cited research project in this area is that of Geoff Pearson – who studied football hooliganism (Pearson, 2011). Pearson (2011) integrated himself into a group of Blackpool F.C. supporters, attending pre-drinks, games, and after-match drinks with them. Pearson's (2011) complete member status allowed him to gain a deeper insight into the behaviours of football fans and crowd disorder. Covert research like Pearson's (2011) is often ethically critiqued for the blurring of boundaries between researcher and complete member. Pearson's involvement in the football fan group led him to commit crimes to strengthen his position within the football fan group and avoid detection as a researcher.

Despite both being complete member researchers, the differences between Pearson's work and the case study are vast. Although both are fully immersed, both acted covertly, and both are participatory, the case study researcher is an opportunistic complete member researcher (Lewis, 2018). This means that before their project, they were already members of the group; their participation within the group is as a member not as a researcher and their covertness is to allow them to continue to be a part of the group after the project is finished. Pearson, on the other hand, was a convert complete member researcher (Kaaristo, 2022); he chose to become a Blackpool fan and match goer to facilitate his research, and his covertness and participation within the group was to maintain his study. Whereas there is a risk (reality) of Pearson going native, the case study researcher is already native, and their indigenousness (through positionality and reflexivity) can be a strength rather than a threat to the qualitative research process (Mason, 2019).

Insider research and complete member research are often linked to feminist methodology. The feminist mantra 'The Personal is Political' has given rise to the 'feminist I' and the use of personal experience and emotions to create evocative and empowering research (Ettorre, 2016). Building on a researcher's positionality not only does feminist research ask us to identify and disclose ourselves to our readers, it goes further to ground our research within our lived experience. In the case study, the researcher has outed themselves as a parent of SEND children, yet we do not know enough about them to know fully how their characteristics might affect the research. Their position as a researcher makes them more powerful than those they are researching, and traditionally this would be considered as something that may affect the dynamic of the project. However, within the case study, the other members of the group are unaware that they are being researched and so will not be affected or influenced by the researcher's existence. When we think about how our characteristics affect research, our gender, race, class, sexuality, and age all can influence our findings. Within online parenting communities, like that of the SEND Facebook group, most active participants have been found to be women and mothers. If the researcher is a man openly interacting with these mothers, he may gain differing data from that of a woman researcher. The elevated levels of education (enough to be conducting a PhD) could also affect the research. SEND parents often feel let down by the system and resultingly are overly critical of professional input, hence why many of them turn to online peer support forums. By outwardly presenting as an academic to these parents, who may already be feeling othered, might cause them to be reluctant to engage with outsiders. Although within the case study the researcher is covertly studying the group, we as readers still do not truly know who the researcher is, and how their life and what they have experienced has influenced the research process and findings. As such, the transparency needed to conduct good qualitative research is limited.

Managing the relationship with the ivory tower
Can subjective disruptive research still be good academic research?
When the voices of the marginalised have been hidden from academic scholarly view due to patriarchal ideals of what counts as knowledge, feminist methods as Black, queer, disabled women push us to challenge the way we research. By placing ourselves in our work, and creating subjective evocative insider research, we can create more authentic, intimate, diverse, and inclusive knowledge (Frances, 2023). By using our own experiences, we can give voice to those going through similar situations, inciting much needed conversations and bringing to the centre those that objective positivist research has pushed to the periphery, knowledge created by us, for us. Despite our similarities and links to those we research, a power differential will always ensue. However, by using our own power, position, and voice to bridge the gap between the ivory tower of academia and the lived realities of those discriminated and ostracised within society, as feminist researchers we can disrupt, and we can create *real* social change (Ettorre, 2017).

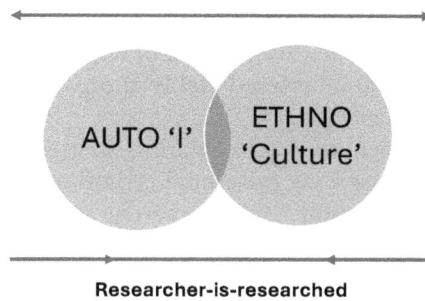

Figure 5.1 Perspectives of autoethnography

When writing about sensitive or taboo topics, researchers are placed in vulnerable positions when asked to declare their positionality. By declaring your personal links to your research, such as depression and suicide, fertility issues and miscarriage, the researcher is labelling themselves to the wider societal readers, colleagues, peers, and future employers. This emotional vulnerability and disclosure can lead to judgement and secondary trauma (Williamson et al, 2020). Within the case study, the researcher's disclosure as being the parent of SEND children not only outs them, but it also outs their children. As social beings, we create and share our identities through conversation and storytelling, but our stories are never just our own. Within each shared narrative are other actors, other people, our loved ones, our friends. The stories that we share not only generate our own identities, but they also reproduce the identities of others, thus raising ethical concerns over consent and confidentiality.

Figure 5.1 is from Doloriert and Sambrook's (2009) paper wherein they describe the auto-ethno/graphic continuum. The model here presents the relationship between our lived experiences as the 'auto' and the broader sociocultural contexts of the 'ethno'.

Not only does our own identity affect how we research, but the context of our research can also affect how we present our identities within our work. Traditionally social science research was written using the third person; this was seen to be more objective – mirroring that of the physical sciences (Badley, 2021). Feminist research has shown how the researcher can place themselves within the research, however still today our academic field, the epistemology of the school in which you are situated and the type of text that is being written, has profound influence on what is deemed *good* research and how this research is presented. From the case study we can see that the researcher is observing and thematically analysing the narratives of other parents (culture), however they are also sharing their own experiences (I), their research flows between the 'auto' and the 'ethno'. When writing journals, or even research method book chapters, the author may be able to distance themselves from the auto, shielding their vulnerability and their nakedness (Meriläinen et al, 2022), but for conferences and the dissemination of their thesis (whereby remaining anonymous causes difficulty in gaining the warranted credit) the author becomes that complete member, embodied within the written and spoken word – laid bare for all to see (Pullen, 2018).

Student voice

My Master's project challenges the use of CTPA in pregnancy. A CTPA is the CT of pulmonary angiogram (PA), the blood vessels in your heart and lungs to see if you have a blood clot. Pregnancy can cause issues with the x-ray dye used during a CTPA, limiting the diagnostic abilities. Despite this, the lack of research into women's health means that often where women could be offered viable alternatives with better results, their needs and experiences are dismissed.

The epistemology of my field means my work is written purely in the third person, and as such I have not disclosed my positionality within my research. I am not even mentioning that I am a radiographer with expertise in the field. My experience as a radiographer shows that most of the doctors pushing for these CTPA are male. My concern is if I place myself in my research, as a woman and mother, my work might not be taken seriously. I may be judged on being a 'hysterical woman' rather than on the quality of my research. As someone who is adamant that women's health is being ignored, I worry that the doctors who need to hear my work will listen better if it came from another man, so by not putting myself in my work I can almost pretend to be one of my male colleagues.

I feel like a lot of the decisions in health made about women's bodies are made by those that are not women, and have never been pregnant. As a female, with two children, I identify with the participants of my study. Although I have never had this procedure, I have been pregnant whilst scanning other pregnant women, and whether I write that in my paper or not still affects my viewpoint.

I have been quite emotional in writing up. From experience I already have a negative view of how people treat women and women's health, I rant about it a lot. I think that if more women were in health research this might change. I went into this research with a motive, I wanted to prove that they were scanning too many pregnant women, a claim that has been argued and ignored many times before. It has been hard when going through the very few bits of data that do not prove my hypothesis, but I must remember that regardless of what my motive is and what I am trying to prove, this is medical research, and I need to be honest with my findings

Conclusion

This chapter has explored how we as researchers manage our relationships with the research, the readers, our participants, and the institution of academia. Feminist methodologies challenge traditional research methods by questioning the fundamental concept of objectivity. Criticising the androcentric bias of traditional research, feminist methods emphasise the inclusion of othered experiences and perspectives to alter the power dynamics in the construction of knowledge and *truth*.

By recognising the social context of social scientific research and writing our own subjectivities into our research, we can break the fourth wall which in turn promotes diverse perspectives, challenges hierarchical and gendered bias inherent in traditional scientific methods, and helps in forming collaborative relationships with both participants and readers.

Recognising that we cannot conduct research objectively opens new avenues for understanding and knowledge production. By embracing our subjectivities, researchers can create more inclusive and meaningful research that reflects the complexity of human life.

In the student's voice section, Hazel wrote about how more women in health research might change the societal view of women's health, yet she still felt it necessary not to position herself within their work. Instead of ignoring our positions and bias, and claiming our work to be objective and scientific, feminists argue we should reject the notion that objective and scientific is the gold standard for scholarly success. We are subjective, emotional, leaking bodies (Pullen, 2018). We all have lived experiences, and our lived experiences matter. Our personal, matters. It is political. Instead of erasing yourself from your work, proudly and loudly place yourself within it. Steer away from the academic tradition that is patriarchal research, write dangerously (Badley, 2021). Use the 'feminist I' (Ettorre, 2016). Use your own voice. After all, we are not all old white men.

Reflective question

How do our understandings of what *good* academic research is challenge the relationship we have with our work, our field, our participants, and our readers?

References

Armstrong, P. (2008) Toward an autoethnographic pedagogy. *Whither Adult Education in the Learning Paradigm*, 43–50.

Badley, GF (2021) We must write dangerously. *Qualitative Inquiry*, 27(6): 716–722.

Boivin, N and CohenMiller, A (2018). Breaking the "fourth wall" in qualitative research: participant-led digital data construction. *Qualitative Report*, 23(3).

Bukamal, H (2022) Deconstructing insider–outsider researcher positionality. *British Journal of Special Education*, 49(3): 327–349.

Cooper, L and Rogers, C (2015) Mothering and 'insider' dilemmas: feminist sociologists in the research process. *British Sociological Association* 20(2). https://doi.org/10.5153/sro.3584

Cuevas-Parra, P (2023) Positionality and reflexivity: recognising and dismantling our privileges in childhood research through the use of windows and mirrors. *Global Studies of Childhood*, 13(4): 295–309.

Deblasio, L (2022) Using reflexivity as a tool to validate feminist research based on personal trauma. *Feminist Legal Studies*, 30(3): 355–365.

Doloriert, C and Sambrook, S (2009) Ethical confessions of the "I" of autoethnography: the student's dilemma. *Qualitative Research in Organizations and Management: An International Journal*, 4(1): 27–45.

Ettorre, E (2016) *Autoethnography as Feminist Method: Sensitising the Feminist 'I'*. Abingdon: Routledge.

Ettorre, E (2017) Feminist autoethnography, gender, and drug use: "feeling about" empathy while "storying the I". *Contemporary Drug Problems*, 44(4): 356–374.

Fenge, L Oakley, L Taylor, B and Beer, S (2019) The impact of sensitive research on the researcher: preparedness and positionality. *International Journal of Qualitative Methods*, 18, 1609406919893161.

Folkes, L (2023) Moving beyond 'shopping list' positionality: using kitchen table reflexivity and in/visible tools to develop reflexive qualitative research. *Qualitative Research*, 23(5): 1301–1318.

Frances, T (2023) Feminist listening and becoming: voice poems as a method of working with young women's stories of domestic abuse in childhood. *Qualitative Research in Psychology*, 20(1): 52–73.

Kaaristo, M (2022) Everyday power dynamics and hierarchies in qualitative research: the role of humour in the field. *Qualitative Research*, 22(5): 743–760.

Karcher, K McCuaig, J and King-Hill, S (2024) (Self-) reflection/reflexivity in sensitive, qualitative research: a scoping review. *International Journal of Qualitative Methods*, 23, 16094069241261860.

Lewis, C (2018) *An Auto-Ethnographic Account of Interactional Practices in Adoptive Family Relationships*. Lancaster University (United Kingdom).

Mason, M (2019) On objectivity and staying 'native': researching LGBTQI+ lawyers as a queer lawyer. In: Creutzfeldt, N Mason, M and McConnachie, K (eds) *Routledge Handbook of Socio-Legal Theory and Methods*. Abingdon: Routledge, pp 123–135.

McNarry, G Allen-Collinson, J and Evans, AB (2024) Somewhere between a stopwatch and a recording device: ethnographic reflections from the pool. *Journal of Contemporary Ethnography*, 53(1): 31–50.

Meriläinen, S Salmela, T and Valtonen, A (2022) Vulnerable relational knowing that matters. *Gender, Work & Organization*, 29(1): 79–91.

Morrow, F and Kettle, M (2024) Putting the auto in ethnography: the embodied process of reflexivity on positionality. *Qualitative Social Work*, 23(3): 554–565.

Pearson, G (2011) *An Ethnography of English Football Fans 1995–2010: Cans, Cops and Carnival*. Manchester: Manchester University Press.

Pullen, A (2018) Writing as labiaplasty. *Organization*, 25(1): 123–130.

Stanley, L and Wise, S (2002) *Breaking Out Again: Feminist Ontology and Epistemology*. Abingdon: Routledge.

Weatherall, R (2023) If on a summer's day a researcher: the implied author and the implied reader in writing differently. *Culture and Organization*, 29(6): 512–527.

Williamson, E et al (2020) Secondary trauma: emotional safety in sensitive research. *Journal of Academic Ethics*, 18: 55–70.

PART II

Designing your research project

CHAPTER 6

Reflective and flexible research

Paula Beesley and Julius Gane

Introduction

Qualitative research is the primary methodology used by health and social care researchers. It can be undertaken using a range of methodologies and methods depending on the researcher's research question, aims and objectives. It takes account of research participants' experiences of a given situation and environmental contexts (Flynn and McDermott, 2016), which requires a reflective, flexible and responsive approach to research participants' needs.

Health and social care research is often undertaken with people, and people are often unpredictable. As such, researchers have to reflect in action to enable them to be responsive to research participants' needs (Berger, 2015; Kara, 2018). Furthermore, reflection in action enables the researcher to acknowledge some of the inequities that are present in many research relationships, which can be addressed through reflective research practice and clear, open communication, and positive, flexible working relationships (Greene, 2014; Flynn and McDermott, 2016).

This chapter provides an overview of reflective and flexible research, specifically looking at how a researcher can reflect *for* ethical and efficient research, react flexibly *in* research to the variances that working with often vulnerable people within health and social care research create, and reflect *on* research processes to enhance research findings. It will conclude with a section reflecting on the needs of people with lived experience who participate in research projects.

Chapter concepts
- Reflective research.
- Making use of a reflective research diary.
- Making use of research supervisors.
- Flexible research within the research process.

DOI: 10.4324/9781041056782-9

Reflective research

Whilst quantitative and scientific researchers argue for the neutrality of the researcher, health and social care research is predominately concerned with understanding positionality within the researcher role and reflectivity of self throughout the study (Greene, 2014). Hence, the focus of positionality in this sense is the researcher's *stance* on the topic created by one's personal and professional values, experiences and educational perspectives (Berger, 2015; Mason-Bish, 2019). Empathic neutrality (Patton, 2015) is achieved by active listening, respect, sensitivity and awareness to demonstrate to the research participant that they are heard and valued. Positionality minimises unconscious bias and enhances the validity of the research outcomes (Mason-Bish, 2019) as Berger notes, 'reflexivity is a major strategy for quality control in qualitative research' (Berger, 2015, p 219). As such, it is recommended that as the chapter progresses a reflective approach is taken to consider personal research reflexivity and flexibility.

Further to this, the researcher should be aware of the research participants' own experiences, using a reflective research approach that acknowledges and considers the impact of self and others on the research outcomes (Braun and Clarke, 2013; Probst and Berenson, 2014; Patton, 2015). From a theoretical perspective, reflective practice for research can be linked to Schön's (1983, 1991) *The Reflective Practitioner*, which suggested that reflection is undertaken in three stages: *reflection for action*, *reflection in action* and *reflection on action*.

First, reflection *for* action concerns the planning stage of a research project. Kara (2018) and Miles et al (2020) argue that an effective researcher makes good use of planning, and whilst that is not to say that they can plan away all obstacles or assume that every ethical dilemma considered prior to undertaking research will arise, reflection in the planning stages can minimise their impact.

This is followed by reflection *in* action, which refers to the flexible responses to the research participants' needs or changes undertaken to respond to real life challenges in data collection or analysis. Ethical dilemmas will occur, and the researcher must weigh up the competing rights and issues to ensure that the most responsible outcome is achieved based on integrity and altruism (Reid et al, 2018), which means working in a trustworthy and reliable manner.

In contrast, reflection *on* action is undertaken after the research activity to consider the impact on the research processes. By taking a step back, the researcher identifies themes in the data that require time for reflection. Interestingly, Pultz (2018) reflected *on* her research with young unemployed people in the Danish welfare system. Pultz (2018) identified how reflection *in action* enhanced her data analysis and research findings. She reflected on the challenges during data collection and her flexible responses to these challenges; thus, clearly indicating how reflection after data collection continues to shape and structure the presenting study.

Space and time should be made to reflect on a regular basis on your research (Olmos-Vega et al, 2022), *in* and *on* action. Whether your research methodology is quantitative or qualitive, or primary or secondary, you should undertake reflection throughout your research project. Here, reflection *for* action will ensure objective data collection is valid and reliable, reflection *in* action will enable you to be flexible in optimising data collection ethically and effectively, and reflection *on* action will ensure your data analysis questions identified themes and evaluates patterns to enhance research findings.

Making use of a reflective research diary

The chapter now considers how a reflective research diary can enhance the research process because it enables active reflection for, in and on action. A research diary enables you to record your thoughts at the time, reflect and develop on them further and return to your reflections with an eye to the critical moments that shaped your research. Probst and Berenson (2014) reflected on the importance of a research diary, which can take the form of post it notes, a diary, field notes, research log, audio recordings or critical incident analysis documents. They recommended daily accounts to note your thoughts on how your research is progressing, as well as reflection for significant events and break through moments, both of which should be returned to and reviewed to enhance your understanding. Whilst there is no absolute requirement of how often to complete a diary entry, it can be helpful to follow a rule of thumb of, for instance, every time a research activity is undertaken to record reflections such as thoughts, feelings, connections. Similarly, style is unimportant; it can be creative (using pictures, diagrams or a stream of consciousness) or structured (using a reflective or critical thinking model). However, key points to include could be:

- Planning ideas, including changes in research question, data collection or analysis method.
- Work undertaken, which will vary depending on the stage of the research project.
- What went well.
- What did not go as well as planned.
- Facts.
- Observations.
- Thoughts and feelings.
- Plans for enhancing the research project.
- Ideas for future consideration, including both for this and future research projects.

Reflective research diaries 'provide a safe forum for students to actively engage with the challenges they experience while taking a research course and take ownership of their learning needs' (Vinjamuri et al, 2017, p 933).

The first purpose of a research diary is to document progress in the research project and as such it can be a factual record, for example:

11 Jan: began literature review, great breadth of existing research available to begin to read.

However, it is more useful to use it as a reflective tool that enables consideration on the research tasks undertaken to develop understanding. For example:

11 Jan: began literature review, great breadth of existing research available to begin to read. After reading a few articles, I realised that I needed to take more comprehensive notes so that I could track each one in the future. I have developed a great chart to complete so that I don't miss anything. It's already paying off because I noticed that some articles cover the method used more robustly than others, which makes me consider reliability of reporting.

Whilst neither is wrong, it is worth considering the purpose of the research diary. If it is to record progress to demonstrate compliance with the research progress, then the simpler approach is sufficient. However, in the second example the reflective approach enabled the researcher to identify an area to develop and action in the form of a chart to ensure equal and comprehensive note taking that would be more useful as the research project developed. Furthermore, the researcher reflected on strengths and weaknesses in published research findings, developing their understanding that they were able to apply to and strengthen their own writing. Importantly, the reflective entry to the research diary enabled the researcher to see an immediate benefit to their research project, which in itself is a reflective action. Overall, the research diary enabled the researcher to track developments, notice themes and patterns, identify areas for development and 'new and exciting modes of enquiry' (Searcey, 2022, pp 187–188), creating multiple benefits beyond the initial reflection.

A reflective research diary should first include reflection *for action*, which will develop accountability for decision-making and enable the defence of research findings if required in the future: why was a questionnaire chosen over an interview; why was participatory research considered appropriate for the research questions; what changes were made as part of this reflective process? Being able to explore initial thoughts and challenges whilst developing a research plan in a reflective research diary aids clarity and understanding of the evidence and personal basis for such decisions (Vinjamuri et al, 2017). A reflective research diary can be used as a form of data collection, reflecting *in action* to note the researcher's thoughts, feelings and responses. The fieldwork diary is particularly useful for an ethnographic methodology where reflective note making on data being collected often identifies unexpected meaning (Searcey, 2022).

Researchers perhaps associate *on action* reflection with experiential learning (Kolb, 1984), where helpful reflective models include Jasper's (2013) ERA model (Experience, Reflection, Action) and Driscoll's (2007) What? model (What? So what? Now what?). Critical thinking models, however, include the five whys model (ask five times 'why' to develop a deeper understanding of the research) or De Bono's (1985) six thinking hats (facts, strengths, restrictions, different ideas, procedures and research ethics, feelings) that enables research practice from a range of perspectives to ensure holistic decision-making which promotes validity and reliability. Using these models as a foundation within a reflective research diary enables the development of research knowledge and skills and will inform changes in the research project. Indeed, Searcey (2022) suggests that returning to reflections can highlight areas missed at the time, thus enhancing your final research outcomes.

A reflective research diary can be solely for the personal use of the researcher or can form the basis of supervision discussion (Vinjamuri et al, 2017). In addition, excerpts from the reflective research diary can be used as part of a research submission, for example a torn diary page insertion can be used to illustrate the reflective research journey (Beesley, 2023).

I found the use of a reflective diary critical to my learning journey as I was able to explore my experiential learning, which in turn developed my research skills. I enhanced this through discussion with my research supervisor, who helped me to identify my strengths and areas for development.

This could be added to the methods section of a research project to supplement a discussion about taking a reflective researcher approach to the project. By including sections of your research diary, you are clearly demonstrating your reflective process and are 'showing your working' as you would in Maths. It can outline and illustrate your reflection for, in and on action and explain your thinking in defence of your research, as inferences made in your research findings can be more clearly seen by your reader or assessor, where they can gain understanding of why you are considering a particular approach or outcome. Finally, inclusion of a research diary will also demonstrate your research skills development, which can be a learning outcome or assessment criteria, so is helpful.

Making use of your research supervisor

Most undergraduate and postgraduate research is undertaken independently, with the guidance of academic teaching and research supervisor support. It seems sensible for students to take as much support as is available to them, as it can only enhance their research skills and their final research report/paper as reflexivity and research outcomes were enhanced through discussion (Probst and Berenson, 2014; Vinjamuri et al, 2017; Olmos-Vega et al, 2022).

Nevertheless, the supervisory relationship is not always easy, and time spent establishing the remit of supervision and expectations can contribute to a successful research supervisory relationship and enhance most research project outcomes (Althubaiti and Althubaiti, 2022). There is an inherent power imbalance in the research supervisory relationship, as the supervisor has knowledge and therefore advice and support that they can choose to impart or withhold. Furthermore, where a supervisor is dogmatic in what the researcher should do, this can limit the ability to be reflective and flexible in developing the research project. Finally, where the research supervisor reviews or grades the final draft of the research dissertation or through cultural hierarchical expectations, the power imbalance can prevent the research participant contributing openly and honestly to supervision discussions. It is recommended that a collaborative approach is undertaken to supervision (Olmos-Vega et al, 2022).

Indeed, collaborative experiential learning (Beesley, 2023) advocates the development of knowledge and skills in supervision through diligence and collaboration. As illustrated in Figure 6.1, both participants attend prepared, having already reflected so that they can engage proactively and effectively. Within supervision the student is empowered to present and discuss ideas which are developed further by the supervisor sharing knowledge and asking open questions to stimulate further reflection.

Often a research supervisor is called a 'critical friend', who is intended to stimulate thinking by asking *provocative questions* from a different perspective than might initially have been considered (Costa and Kallick, 1993). A critical friend can be structured – a set amount of appointments with a clearly defined agenda and expectations for each supervision – or a less formal, often ad hoc arrangement – perhaps a chat over a coffee to explore a problem. Both are equally valid and effectively support reflective thinking (MacPhail et al, 2024). Irrespective, research students should be challenged and supported into and through their zone of proximal development (Vygotsky, 1978), as discussed in Chapter 4, which is the gap between current skills and potential

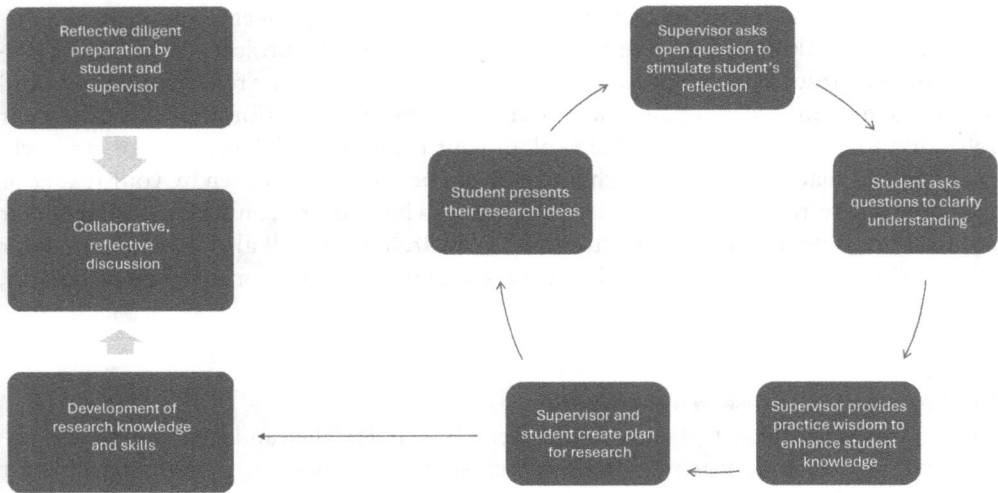

Figure 6.1 Collaborative experiential learning

ability to learn with support. Indeed, Costa and Kallick (1993) argued that engaging reflectively with a critical friend nurtured open-mindedness and therefore a flexible approach to research and research skill development.

However, research students need to be open to feedback, both positive and constructive criticism. Carless and Boud (2018) argued that feedback literacy is achieved where students value and understand the value of feedback, can reflect on their own strengths and areas for development through internal feedback, are able to manage their feelings about feedback and are able to reflect on and action feedback given by others. It can be difficult to *hear* feedback and research students are required to have a reflective approach to enable them to hear and action feedback to develop research skills and enhance areas for development. It is here that the benefit of a reflective research diary entry is returned to. If a contemporaneous diary entry is made, this ensures that the collaborative experiential learning loop is completed as the students reflect on the feedback and use the reflective writing exercise to further develop and embed their enhanced research practice. Indeed, an initial defensive response to feedback can often be meliorated by time and the reflective mirror created in a diary entry. Indeed, Olmos-Vega et al (2022, p 241) define reflexivity as 'a set of continuous, collaborative, and multifaceted practices through which researchers self-consciously critique, appraise, and evaluate how their subjectivity and context influence the research processes'.

Flexible research

Lincoln and Guba (1985, p 42) refer to trustworthiness as 'validity, reliability and objectivity'. Quantitative and scientific research reliability comes from structure, consistency and uniformity. In contrast, qualitative research's reliability, and therefore strength, arguably comes from its flexibility (Billo and Hiemstra, 2013; McArdle, 2022), as 'this is not a loss or a narrowing of ideas but an opening up, using an alternative lens' (McArdle, 2022, p 625).

Flexible research is the ability to respond to the situation, adapt the research plan to cope with uncertainty and change and to meet the presented needs of the research project. It requires critical thinking, often to weigh up the competing needs of the situation and to make a decision based on research ethics, procedural requirements and research participants' needs. In health and social care, qualitative researchers often work with vulnerable people with lived experience and need to be responsive to ensure that they remain person-centred rather than procedurally orientated. However, this illustrates an important point in flexible research: it should not be spontaneous and reactive without being reflective, as the researcher still needs to defend their decision-making to ensure the research outcomes remain valid and reliable.

McArdle (2022) argued that using qualitative methodologies creates multiple opportunities which demands a flexible and responsive approach. However, she developed this further by arguing for the importance of planning for flexibility so that researchers could predict potential pitfalls. Indeed, she argued that by anticipating the challenges and planning for a flexible research plan that has structure but equally allows for unexpected events to occur, the research project will be easier to navigate and ultimately more effective.

Flexibility can also engage research participants. The approach of locating data collection where the research participants are naturally located has two clear advantages: first that participants may feel more comfortable in their surroundings, and second that the period required to participate is shorter as they do not need to travel to the site of the research (Miles et al, 2020). Qualitative research often advocates the use of flexible data collection, for example the use of a semi-structured interview or focus group enables flexible responses to research participants. It can therefore be helpful to plan regular review points to ensure that the research project remains relevant and appropriate.

It is helpful to locate flexible research in health, social care and social work, as this is an arena with diverse health and disability issues. An **AWE** research approach can be considered, where there is an:

Awareness about the research terrain and the research participants' needs, that leads to an ethical plan that incorporates the liberty to

Wiggle and provide necessary adjustments to original data collection plans to facilitate the

Execution of data collection that incorporates necessary adjustments which will enable the researcher to work towards a reliable research outcome.

The AWE concept advocates that health and social care researchers value reflexivity and flexibility, bearing in mind or valuing the 'nature' of its research participants – they may be impacted by health issues, capacity issues or even by the ability to engage due to timing or meeting environment. The onus therefore lies on the researcher to uphold the integrity of the research output and predict, respond to and understand the necessary modifications required for the benefit of ethical research outcomes.

Data analysis should be undertaken with an open mind and flexible response using an inductive approach (Engel and Schutt, 2017) to ensure that pre-conceived notions are not identified and ratified through a biased approach. It is not unusual to find unexpected research findings, which are only seen by the researcher where they are flexible and reflective. In contrast, researchers may have to be flexible in discarding or combining initial themes where there is insufficient or inconsistent evidence (Braun and

Clarke, 2006). Finally, the presentation of research findings should be written 'creatively and with some flair' (Yin, 2018, p 220). Flynn and McDermott (2016) emphasise the importance of writing findings for a wider audience, so that the research has an impact, meaning that a flexible approach should be taken to engage the audience and may be different if it is for a journal article, academic paper or feedback for service users.

Research should be flexible, problem solving, person-centred and responsive to enable ethical research that does no harm but is able to engage often vulnerable people with lived experience in a reflective and flexible manner (Kara, 2018) (see Chapters 7 and 8). The researcher should therefore have an ethical attitude and remain 'morally active' (McLaughlin, 2012, p 71), which requires a reflective and flexible approach.

Student voice

As a social work apprentice, this reflection considers my personal experience gained through engagement, assessment and support planning with adults that have complex physical and mental health and/or disability needs and those who are experiencing homelessness. Working with vulnerable people requires us to be flexible, responsive and often creative, and undertaking research with vulnerable people requires the same approach. Horner (2019) identified, for example, that a person with a learning disability has borne the attributes of social and personal vulnerabilities associated with impairment of cognition and their experiences of oppression. This may affect engagement, communication and understanding, so how might planning a conventional research project impact data collection with such a person?

Saliya (2023) has identified that conventional research methods – following a sequential data collection, smooth analytical technique and interpretations – should not always be the ideal approach in every research situation and that there can be a role for flexibility in research. In health, social care and social work (or social research), data is gathered from people to inform policy, law and legislation, and must therefore engender an approach to uphold the value of reliability.

Ethical scrutiny and approval are required under the Mental Capacity Act 2005 for vulnerable adults to participate in research (Parker et al, 2011), which also reinforces the vital role for flexibility in research in health, social care and social work. It might be obvious, but ethical approval for researchers can demonstrate an act of respect and appropriateness towards dignity in any research planning, especially within the health, social care and social work arena. Researchers must be able to adjust plans to work towards an expected research outcome – a step that creates a role for flexibility in research, for example planning a contingency plan where they anticipate that potential research participants may not be consistently able or available to engage in research projects, as they may not adhere to the strict timescale of a research plan or Gantt chart requirements. This creates a need for flexibility for the sake of greater research engagement.

To conclude, the health, social care and social work arena largely comprises vulnerable people – with various or complex learning, health and life challenging issues. As such, conducting research within this terrain will require the need to adopt flexible strategies that can work in achieving a reliable outcome from any piece of research. The AWE research approach can therefore be considered when researchers are planning their work within this terrain.

Conclusion

Reflection is a core skill for health and social care students, and professionals' skill enhances practice and confidence. When applied to research it is equally as important as it enhances research practice, confidence and research outcomes. By reflecting *for action* in the planning stage, researchers can envisage problems and flexibly adjust ethical approval and research proposals to enhance data collection and data analysis methods. However, it is impossible to anticipate all issues that will arise as health and social care research is often undertaken with vulnerable research participants and researchers need to reflect *in action* to enable them to respond flexibly to arisen needs. Finally, researchers should allocate time to reflect *on action* to enhance their data analysis as they flexibly see themes emerging by considering the data analysis codes that have arisen.

The chapter has reflected on the constructive use of a reflective research diary and a research supervisor, both of which enhance your understanding of research practice and enhance your research knowledge and skills. It is by taking a reflective and flexible approach that takes account of research processes and research participants' needs that qualitative health and social care research becomes ethical, valid and reliable. Any flexible adjustments can be made provisional that they are outlined and justified within the research report or paper to ensure accountability and transparency by the researcher.

Reflective questions

1. Do you reflect on your practice on a regular basis? If so, transfer your reflective skills to the development of your research skills.
2. Do you feel that reflection is a challenge to your practice and research skills? If so, consider how you can enhance your reflection skills with your research supervisor.
3. Do you feel open to being a flexible researcher, how do you cope with and respond to change?
4. How do you feel about reflection and flexibility as ways of achieving unexpected research findings and how might you embrace these in your research skills development?

References

Althubaiti, A and Althubaiti, S (2022) Medical research: what to expect in a student–supervisor relationship. *BMC Medical Education*, 22(1): article 774.

Beesley, P (2023) Collaborative experiential learning in social work practice placements. *Social Work Education*, 1–16.

Berger, R (2015) Now I see it, now I don't: researcher's position and reflexivity in qualitative research. *Qualitative Research*, 15(2): 219–234.

Billo, E and Hiemstra, N (2013) Mediating messiness: expanding ideas of flexibility, reflexivity, and embodiment in fieldwork. *Gender, Place and Culture*, 20(3): 313–328.

Braun, V and Clarke, V (2006) Using thematic analysis in psychology. *Qualitative Research in Psychology*, 3(2): 77–101.

Braun, V and Clarke, V (2013) *Successful Qualitative Research. A Practical Guide for Beginners*. London: Sage.

Carless, D and Boud, D (2018) The development of student feedback literacy: enabling uptake of feedback. *Assessment & Evaluation in Higher Education*, 43(8): 1315–1325.

Costa, A and Kallick, B (1993) Through the lens of a critical friend. *Educational Leadership*, 51(2): 49–51.

De Bono, E (1985) *Six Thinking Hats*. Boston: Little Brown and Company.

Driscoll, J (2007) Supported reflective learning: the essence of clinical supervision. In: Driscoll, J (ed) *Practising Clinical Supervision: A Reflective Approach for Healthcare Professionals.* Edinburgh: Balliere Tindall, pp 27–51.

Engel, R and Schutt, R (2017) *The Practice of Research in Social Work*. London: Sage.

Flynn, C and McDermott, F (2016) *Doing Research in Social Work and Social Care. The Journey form Student to Practitioner Researcher*. London: Sage.

Greene, M (2014) On the inside looking in: methodological insights and challenges in conducting qualitative insider research. *The Qualitative Report*, 19(29): 1–13.

Horner, N (2019) *What is Social Work? Contexts and Perspectives*. 5th Edn. London: Learning Matters.

Kara, H (2018) *Research Ethics in the Real World*. Bristol: Policy Press.

Kolb, D (1984) *Experiential Learning: Experience as the Source of Learning and Development*. (Vol. 1). New Jersey: Prentice-Hall.

Lincoln, Y and Guba, E (1985) *Naturalistic Inquiry*. London: Sage.

MacPhail, A, Tannehill, D and Ataman, R (2024) The role of the critical friend in supporting and enhancing professional learning and development. *Professional Development in Education*, 50(4): 597–610.

Mason-Bish, M (2019) The elite delusion: reflexivity, identity and positionality in qualitative research. *Qualitative Research*, 19(3): 263–276.

McArdle, R (2022) Flexible methodologies: A case for approaching research with fluidity. *The Professional Geographer*, 74(4): 620–627.

McLaughlin, H (2012) *Understanding Social Work Research*. London: Sage.

Miles, M, Huberman, M and Saldana, J (2020) *Qualitative Data Analysis: A Methods Sourcebook*. London: Sage.

Olmos-Vega, F, Stalmeijer, R, Varpio, L and Kahlke, R (2022) A practical guide to reflexivity in qualitative research: AMME Guide No. 149. *Medical Teacher*, 45(3): 241–251.

Parker, J, Penhale, B and Stanley D (2011) Research ethics review: social care and social science research and the Mental Capacity Act 2005. *Ethics and Social Welfare*, 5(4): 380–400.

Patton, M (2015) *Qualitative Research and Evaluation Methods*. London: Sage.

Probst, B and Berenson, L (2014) The double arrow: how qualitative social work researchers use reflexivity. *Qualitative Social Work*, 13(6): 813–827.

Pultz, S (2018) Flexibility in research design: how unexpected events can improve learning and research. *SAGE Research Methods Cases*. London: SAGE Publications.

Reid, A, Brown, J, Smith, J, Cope, A and Jamieson, S (2018) Ethical dilemmas and reflexivity in qualitative research. *Perspectives on Medical Education*, 7(2): 69–75.

Saliya, C (2023) Integrated-flexible research methodology: an alternative approach. In: Saliya, C (ed) *Social Research Methodology and Publishing Results: A Guide to Non-Native English Speakers*. USA: IGI Global, pp 1–10.

Schön, D (1983) *The Reflective Practitioner*. London: Maurice Temple Smith.

Schön, D (1991) *The Reflective Practitioner*. London: Ashgate.

Searcey, R (2022) Capturing accidental moments: the self-reflective researcher and the utility of the research diary. In: Sanders, T, McGarry, K and Ryan, P (eds) *Sex Work, Labour and Relations*. London: Palgrave Macmillan, pp 185–208.

Vinjamuri, M, Warde, B and Kolb, P (2017) The reflective diary: an experiential tool for enhancing social work students' research learning. *Social Work Education*, 36(8): 933–945.

Vygotsky, LS (1978) *Mind in Society: The Development of Higher Psychological Process*. Cambridge MA: Harvard University Press.

Yin, R (2018) *Case Study Research and Applications*. Design and methods. California: Sage.

CHAPTER 7

Including vulnerable participants in research

Chloe Blackwell, Carrie Harrop and Matt Padley

Introduction

Involving people from vulnerable groups in research, which purports to represent issues affecting them, is important for research validity (its 'truth' and trustworthiness in explaining phenomena), and it avoids overlooking or misrepresenting their perspectives. The principle of 'nothing about us, without us' is a critical one in research with vulnerable groups, emphasising the need to, and importance of, include vulnerable participants in research relating to or focused on their experiences of and positions within the world. However, many researchers worry about including vulnerable people in research because of the potential challenges that it can raise. In a practical sense, it can be difficult to find participants. Researchers often need the support of others to gain access to vulnerable, hard-to-reach groups; non-government organisations, local authorities or parents can become 'gatekeepers' to recruitment and research. Thinking about the position of vulnerable participants can raise ethical questions about the best approaches to including them in research.

Research in health and social care often aims to understand and improve the experiences of vulnerable and marginalised groups. In a general sense, groups are understood as vulnerable if they are at increased relative risk of harm and/or experience diminished autonomy. Meanwhile, for the purpose of research and ethics, there exist contesting conceptualisations of vulnerability which Gordon (2020) says can be placed into two groups: (1) the categorical approach and (2) the contextual approach. The categorical approach is more rigid, identifying whole groups or characteristics as vulnerable, while the contextual approach views vulnerability as more variable, depending on each person and the situation they are in. Authors like Aldridge (2016) and Liamputtong (2007) have demonstrated that vulnerability is relative rather than fixed, situated in the time and place in which a person lives. Understanding vulnerability in this way, people are not inherently vulnerable because of their characteristics or experiences, but because of the ways that society treats particular individuals or groups. The social and cultural context can generate vulnerability via processes of discrimination. Research, too, is

DOI: 10.4324/9781041056782-10

part and parcel of the social context. In covering topics related to the lives of vulnerable groups, it can highlight the issues they face and challenge them. However, research also has the potential to reproduce marginalisation (for example, through harmful ways of describing people or negative framing of experiences), and this is especially a risk if the research excludes vulnerable participants.

Chapter concepts

This chapter makes a case for the inclusion of vulnerable participants in research, and it describes some of the ways that this can be done. The following key concepts inform discussions throughout:

- Power and positionality: of researchers, participants and gatekeepers
- Participant choice and capacity
- Ethical research design and practice

> **Reflective question**
>
> As you read this chapter, take some time to reflect on your own experiences of working with vulnerable individuals or groups. How can we make sure that research with these groups respects and reflects their lived experiences?

Vulnerability and research participation

Good research design will carefully consider its study population (that is, which participants to include in the study). The inclusion criteria for the study population will typically be shaped by questions, one of which is: what participant characteristics and experiences will be relevant to the study's research questions and aims? The study may require that participants are of a particular gender, ethnicity, place of residence, age or life stage (i.e., of school or pension age) or occupation (e.g., a teacher, therapist or prison officer). Often, answering a set of research questions will also require that the study population has experience of certain relationships (e.g., they are a parent, sibling or spouse), or that they possess specific life experiences (e.g., experience of the care system). People considered vulnerable may have key experiences relevant to a particular study. A UK study, for example, which aimed to understand the impact of the Covid-19 pandemic on the wellbeing of adults with learning disabilities prioritised interviews with adults with learning disabilities (Flynn et al, 2021). In another study, 48 interviews with imprisoned women were combined with participant observation to explore staff–prisoner relationships (Crewe et al, 2023).

Another question influencing the inclusion and, perhaps more specifically, *exclusion* criteria of a study is this: what are the potential harms that involvement in research could cause to different participants? People from vulnerable groups may have already experienced trauma, discrimination and physical or psychological abuse, and there may be the concern that their involvement in research would risk exposing them to further marginalisation or distress. This is the point where vulnerable groups may be excluded from research, because although their experiences would make them knowledgeable participants, there may also be a (real or perceived) higher level of associated risk. Something which may be overlooked when thinking about risk is that participants are not passive in the recruitment and research process. With the right information, presented at an appropriate level, participants can weigh up the risks and benefits of research, and whether participation is right or not will vary from individual to individual. When asked about research participation, a group of adults with intellectual and developmental disabilities, for example, said they saw it as a valuable and important way of informing understanding and policy on issues relevant to their lives (McDonald et al, 2013).

A research team or ethics board may have concerns that people from vulnerable groups would be unable to contribute to a study because they do not possess the capacity to understand or answer questions. There may be assumptions around the mental capacity of, for example, children, the elderly, people with alcohol or substance abuse disorder, people with dementia, people with poor mental health or people with learning disabilities. Mental capacity, just like vulnerability, is not a straightforward issue. Assumptions about the mental capacity of others can be wrong, mental capacity is not a fixed state (people's mental capacity can vary over time) and even where a person is found not to have the mental capacity to give their legal consent to research, this does not necessarily mean that they cannot participate. Research guidance informed by the Mental Capacity Act 2005 promotes the inclusion of vulnerable participants, stipulating that a person should be assumed to have the mental capacity (to retain information and/or give informed consent) until they demonstrate otherwise (see King's College Hospital, no date; NHS Health Research Authority, 2021). Under the Mental Capacity Act 2005, being found to lack capacity *does not* lead to the automatic exclusion of a person from activities such as research. Rather, the act places a responsibility on professionals (including researchers), advocates and consultees to work with the person to consider what inclusion should look like and to explore ways that the person can participate without it becoming disproportionately onerous. Children under the age of 16 (a group that regularly has their mental capacity for research questioned) do not come under the Mental Capacity Act 2005, and they cannot give legal informed consent, rather consent is provided by an adult, and the child participant provides their assent (their agreement) to take part in the research.

Another question which may influence the final study population is this: Is it feasible and practical to include participants from certain groups? Research with vulnerable groups may, for example, require more time to prepare materials. Participants may need research information and consent forms in different formats, such as in braille, in another language or in an easy-read layout. In preparing for research, researchers may also need more time with participants to build rapport, trust or to gain an understanding of the participant's communication style and needs. The challenge of recruiting people from vulnerable groups can also be a barrier to their participation in research. Researchers often need to rely on connections built with organisations, including charities and community groups, or with institutions, such as prisons and schools, to reach vulnerable groups. Recruiting participants through 'gatekeepers' such as these can be highly useful, but it can also involve a lot of negotiation (see later in this chapter for further discussion).

Given the various potential challenges, student and academic researchers may opt to exclude vulnerable groups from their study. They may choose instead to gather information about vulnerable groups *by proxy*, for example interviewing parents or school staff to understand the experiences of children, talking to people working in homeless shelters to learn about the needs of people without homes or talking to professional care workers to understand the experiences of people who use their services. The decision to exclude a vulnerable group from research is problematic, especially if it has been made without consulting anyone who represents that group. Recruiting proxy participants and not potentially vulnerable participants may be rationalised on ethical grounds, and yet the exclusion itself can further marginalise vulnerable groups. Hill et al (2004, p 77) pointed out that many initiatives impacting the lives of children, for example, have been 'designed, delivered and evaluated by adults'. Making a study easier to carry out is not in and of itself an adequate rationale for excluding potentially vulnerable research participants. Research overall should include the full range of viewpoints and pay careful attention to the balance of voices being represented.

Researchers at all career stages benefit from support, and this can be especially important for studies with vulnerable participants. In designing a study, literature on methods and ethics is a good place to start. A lot can be learned too from the process of making an application to an ethics committee, something which is necessary for beginning any research with participants (see Chapter 4). Researcher support should also continue throughout a study. Shaw et al (2019), in a paper including case studies of students conducting research with vulnerable groups, recommended that in addition to ethics training, new researchers benefit from mentorship and peer support, which gives them the opportunity to discuss hypothetical risks and responses as well as to debrief and reflect on fieldwork already carried out. The next section presents different considerations for the design and conduct of research which includes participants from vulnerable groups. Chapter 9 also includes a focused discussion on research and planning.

Research with vulnerable participants

This section introduces the ways that research can include vulnerable participants, organised into two key aspects of qualitative studies: (1) research design, and (2) recruitment and fieldwork.

Research design

There are certain things that researchers in the UK must do when conducting research that involves vulnerable participants, such as completing a criminal background check (a Disclosure and Barring Service check in England and Wales) and applying for ethical clearance from an appropriate ethical committee. Beyond these 'procedural ethics' (Shiraani et al, 2022), researchers have some choice around how they approach research design. It is understandable that researchers can find themselves in a 'comfort zone' with particular research methods, especially when those methods are well-established. Student researchers may be drawn to methods which are widely practised and therefore often written about. However, studies with vulnerable participants may require researchers to think more creatively about the methods they use, because what is comfortable for the researcher will not necessarily be comfortable or beneficial for the participants. It might be more useful to use photography or videos, diaries or drawings, for example (see Kara, 2015), rather than approaches that can feel more formal, such as traditional interviews or focus groups. Flexibility in methodological approaches is highly valuable in research conducted with vulnerable participants too. See also Chapter 10 for more on qualitative research discussions, and Chapter 11 for detail on creative approaches.

Even where studies use more traditional methods, vulnerable participants might feel more comfortable taking part in research if they can choose between different ways to participate, for example, interviewing over the phone, face-to-face or online. A study may also offer participants the choice between responding to research questions synchronously (answering questions in real-time) or asynchronously (answering questions over a longer period through online forums with other participants or one-to-one over email with the researcher). Research flexibility may also extend to the spaces used to conduct research, and the researcher can consult participants about whether to conduct research in a real or virtual space or in a private (such as the participant's home) or public space (such as in a community centre). Thinking about the possible impact of different spaces on participants is important. For example, although a study on foster care may benefit from access to a room with the council to conduct interviews, this may not be an appropriate location for interviewees who have experienced foster care. Conducting research and data collection online has become more prevalent, especially in response to the Covid-19 pandemic, and yet this method will not be suitable for a study population who are likely to be digitally excluded. You can find more on research flexibility in Chapter 6.

There are many options for including a variety of participants in research, but ultimately the researcher must make a choice about which approach(es) to use. Drawing on the advice and expertise of others is a key part of designing and developing research, and it is especially important where studies are including a typically overlooked study population. A good place to start is with a review of the existing literature as this is where academics and student researchers can draw on what others have learned (theoretically, methodologically and ethically) in conducting research in a similar field. It is also beneficial to consult non-academic experts for the development of research. Researchers can call on the advice of people working in institutions (such as schools), third sector organisations (such as charities or community organisations) and people with lived experience (including people from vulnerable groups). There are different ways that these experts can get involved in research too. A study may organise paid or unpaid advisory groups, comprising a range of non-academic experts. Alternatively, researchers with fewer resources may approach advisors more informally. In whichever way advisors are consulted, it is typically the case that researchers will ultimately decide on the design of the study. In contrast, co-production in research means that non-academic experts become more involved in a study, playing a key role in the decision making involved in the research design, analysis and writing (Aldridge, 2016; Power et al, 2024). Research may also involve one or several *peer researchers* who are a part of the community being studied, such as an elderly community, a neurodiverse community or a community living in a particular location.

Recruitment and fieldwork

There are other instances, aside from advisory groups, where a study may call on a variety of professionals or consultees (e.g., family members). They can help with the recruitment of participants who are, perhaps due to their position of vulnerability, difficult to identify or access. Family members may provide legal consent on behalf of the participant, for example if the participant is under the age of 16, or they may act as an advisor for research with participants who do not have the mental capacity to give informed consent at the time of fieldwork. Professionals, advocates and family members of participants who aid research in these ways play an important role as a mutual point of contact and support for researchers and potential participants. As 'gatekeepers' they also influence who is recruited for research and the type and extent of researcher–participant interaction that takes place, and thereby hold a position of power. As the first point of contact, gatekeepers can make participation decisions on behalf of others, potentially without consulting the people that the research aims to recruit. This can mean that potential participants have not necessarily had the opportunity to consider their involvement in research and what that might mean for them, or inversely that participants put forward for research may have been coerced into doing so. It is best practice to go through the participant information with all participants, and never to assume that gatekeepers or any third party has passed on all the information. As in all research, monitoring consent and assent of participants is an ongoing process and does not end with the participant completing the ethics paperwork (see Hart et al, 2020). See Chapter 4 for more discussion of ethics.

Professionals, family members and carers of vulnerable participants may take part in the research themselves, synchronously or asynchronously, perhaps because the research aims to understand a phenomenon from multiple perspectives, or perhaps to better enable people from vulnerable groups to participate. For example, some participants may feel more able and comfortable to take part in research if they can do so alongside a trusted person who knows them well. Including different perspectives and 'voices' presents ethical questions, such as how the research will deal with potential power imbalances. Researchers may need to think about how they will conduct research where some participants might be more likely to share their views (and have their views heard) than others. As part of this, they may consider the extent to which their selected approaches can help them redress the imbalance of 'voices'? In synchronous methods, vulnerable participants may be quick to withdraw an expressed opinion when it is challenged by a co-participant in a higher position of power. When disagreement occurs between participants, a possible researcher response is to remain quiet in a bid to maintain neutrality (Valentine, 1999; Zarhin, 2018), or sometimes it may be more appropriate for the researcher to be more active in the conversation to facilitate it and elevate the viewpoints of less dominant speakers (Evens & Houssart, 2007). Chapters 4 and 5 provide more detail on issues around power and relationships.

Student voice

As someone who grew up in the English foster care system, my experience has influenced how and why I conduct research. I have embraced the concept of being a 'peer researcher' (someone who draws on their lived experiences to conduct research), rather than trying to remove or ignore my connections to the topics I choose to research. I have been open about my background in the care system during recruitment and data collection, something which I consider to be a strength. Carrying out research as a peer researcher has meant that I have had to be very aware of my position and I have had to pay special attention to particular aspects of research.

Being aware of the potential risks and ethical issues before you carry out your research is paramount, which is why the ethics process for working with vulnerable participants often requires more in-depth consideration and information. Spending quality time on your ethics application will help to ensure that your research is not compromised by not acknowledging potential risks and ethical considerations at panel. Taking into consideration the areas above within the application will help to ensure that you are not caught off guard or having to go through the ethical approval process again.

As a student researcher you may be more likely to research an area in which you are already connected, and as such be a peer researcher. If this is the case, then the additional considerations around vulnerabilities and ethics should be considered, as it will likely be an area of further work when going through the ethics process and when carrying out the research. For example, as a student researcher (and beyond) looking after your own mental health while carrying out research is key. You may wish to consider approaching the mental health services within the university or externally to ensure you can process the information and data collected during the research without it having a negative impact on yourself.

Even if you are not a peer researcher, ensuring support is in place when working with vulnerable groups is recommended as it is likely you will be researching and collecting data that could potentially cause harm to you as a researcher, but also to the participants, if not carried out in a well thought out, and trauma informed way. Ensuring the safety of all of those involved in research is important for any research, however when considering research with participants who may be facing more vulnerabilities, this becomes a key area for consideration.

It might be helpful to reach out to external organisations who can provide support to participants, for example mental health support, or advocacy support. If you are interviewing a participant about their own experiences of difficult and potentially traumatic experiences, ensuring support is available is paramount when considering the potential risks and ethical consequences and considerations. For example, if you are interviewing or carrying out research in person, you must consider the potential risks and ensure that well thought out risk assessments are completed. Even if meeting virtually, you must work to protect yourself as a researcher and the participants.

Looking after yourself as a researcher should always be considered; for example, you are not feeling on top form, or if you feel that the content of the data you are collecting is causing you upset, step back, speak to your supervisor/s and outside support and reassess the situation. This might mean ending an interview early, or taking a step back from your data set to ensure you are looking after your wellbeing. These additional considerations should not mean you do not carry out research with participants facing additional vulnerabilities, it just means you need to take on deeper processes of ethical considerations and personal reflection.

Conclusion

Good research in social care, and in social science more broadly, gives voice to and illuminates the full range of viewpoints, experiences, relationships and structures which combine to make up the social world. Research with vulnerable groups has a key role to play, highlighting the issues that certain groups may face, and, at its best, working with participants to co-produce knowledge, understanding and ultimately change. The 'nothing about us, without us' principle is key in research with vulnerable individuals and groups.

Working with vulnerable participants will not always be possible – there are undoubtedly circumstances where any potential benefits of research rightly take second place to the potential distress or harm that various research practices and processes could bring. But where it is possible to include vulnerable groups, it is doubly important that we as students and practitioners involved in research are even more acutely aware of our responsibilities to those we are doing research with. This starts with reflecting on our own position/s and power and how this relates to the position and power of participants. It continues through privileging ethical concerns, developing robust ethical frameworks centred on informed consent, anonymity and confidentiality, underpinned by an ongoing duty and ethics of care. It should shape how we do research – flexibility in methodological approaches, adaptable and accommodating in when, where and how research takes place. And in communicating what we have found, we should focus on ensuring accessibility. For all involved – vulnerable individuals and groups, students, practitioners, universities and society – there is so much to be gained from doing ethically robust research that offers the opportunity to deepen and grow our understanding and knowledge, to inform change.

Reflective questions

1. Reflect on your learning through this chapter. How has this affected your thinking about working with vulnerable individuals and/or groups?
2. What are the challenges you face in your practice or research in working with vulnerable participants?
3. What support do you think you would benefit from in working with vulnerable participants? Can you identify where you might find this support?

References

Aldridge, J (2016) *Participatory Research: Working with Vulnerable Groups in Research and Practice*. Bristol: Policy Press.

Crewe, B Schliehe, A and Przybylska, DA (2023) 'It causes a lot of problems': relational ambiguities and dynamics between prisoners and staff in a women's prison. *European Journal of Criminology*, 20(3): 925–946.

Evens, H and Houssart, J (2007) Paired interviews in mathematics education. *BSRLM Proceedings*, 27(2). Available at: https://bsrlm.org.uk/publications/proceedings-of-day-conference/ip27-2/

Flynn, S Hayden, N Clarke, L Caton, S Hatton, C Hastings, R Abbott, D Beyer, S Bradshaw, J Gillooly, A Gore, N Heslop, P Jahoda, A Maguire, R Marriott, A Oloidi, E Paris, A Mulhall,

P Scior, K... Todd, S (2021) *Coronavirus and People with Learning Disabilities Study, Wave 3 Results.* University of Warwick.

Gordon, BG (2020) Vulnerability in research: basic ethical concepts and general approach to review. *Ochsner Journal*, 20(1): 34–38.

Hart, SM Pascucci, M Sood, S and Barrett, EM (2020) Value, vulnerability and voice: an integrative review on research assent. *British Journal of Learning Disabilities*, 48(2): 154–161.

Hill, M Davis, J Prout, A and Tisdall, K (2004) Moving the participation agenda forward. *Children & Society*, 18(2): 77–96.

Kara, H (2015) *Creative Research Methods in the Social Sciences: A Practical Guide.* Bristol: Policy Press.

King's College Hospital (no date) *Research Department Capacity and Research – Guidance for Researchers.* Available at: www.kch.nhs.uk/document/mental-capacity-act-mca-for-researchers/ (accessed 11 September 2024).

Liamputtong, P (2007) *Researching the Vulnerable.* London: SAGE Publications.

McDonald, KE Kidney, CA and Patka, M (2013) 'You need to let your voice be heard': research participants' views on research. *J Intellect Disabil Res*, 57(3): 216–225.

Mental Capacity Act 2005, c9.

NHS Health Research Authority (2021) *Mental Capacity Act.* Available at: www.hra.nhs.uk/planning-and-improving-research/policies-standards-legislation/mental-capacity-act/ (accessed 11 September 2024).

Shaw, RM Howe, J Beazer, J and Carr, T (2019) Ethics and positionality in qualitative research with vulnerable and marginal groups. *Qualitative Research*, 20(3): 277–293.

Shiraani, F Shaheer, I and Carr, N (2022) Procedural ethics vs being ethical: a critical appraisal. In: Okumus, F Rasoolimanesh, SM and Jahani, S (eds) *Contemporary Research Methods in Hospitality and Tourism.* Leeds: Emerald Publishing Limited, pp 21–37.

Power, M, Patrick, R and Garthwaite, K (2024) "I feel like I am part of something bigger than me": methodological reflections from longitudinal online participatory research. *International Review of Qualitative Research.*

Valentine, G (1999) Doing household research: interviewing couples together and apart. *Area*, 31(1): 67–74.

Zarhin, D (2018) Conducting joint interviews with couples: ethical and methodological challenges. *Qualitative Health Research*, 28(5): 844–854.

Involvement of people with lived experiences in research

Amy Payne, Lorne Power, Mandy Simpson, Cynthia Tuuli and Kay Wall

Introduction

'Should research be conducted on people or with people?'

This chapter will explore this statement and build on earlier chapters regarding ethical considerations within the research process. It will challenge you to reflect on traditional research approaches and the power dynamics that exist between the researcher and those who are 'researched'. Current policy changes will be explored that have necessitated the need for people with lived experience (PWLE) to be more fully involved in the research process. This contrasts with traditional academic-led research, where the researcher holds all the decision-making power with PWLE involvement viewed purely as participants. Examples and case studies will be used throughout the chapter to highlight fundamental principles to guide you as you consider your research proposal.

Participatory, inclusive, and co-produced research are all forms of collaborative research that aim to engage people with a lived experience in research. It moves away from the notion of research *on* people to research conducted *with* people (Nind, 2017). Moreover, it draws on personal experience and the generating of knowledge together with PWLE, rather than extracting information from PWLE (Nind and Vinha, 2014; Nind, 2017; John et al, 2018). For collaborative research, the research must be meaningful to the individuals being studied, clearly represent their views and experiences, and treat PWLE who take part in research with respect (John et al, 2018; Nind, 2017). PWLE can be involved in research in a variety of ways. They can act as advisors, be involved as co-researchers, or even lead and conduct their own research on topics that are important to them. In these examples, PWLE contribute their skills and experience and generate new knowledge perspectives (Bigby et al, 2014; Puyalto et al, 2016; Levac et al, 2019). The important principle that needs to be highlighted is that PWLE are offered the opportunity to contribute to the research in a way that is appropriate and meaningful for that individual, and the nature of the research project. This will be explored throughout the chapter.

DOI: 10.4324/9781041056782-11

Chapter concepts
- Valuing individuals
- Enabling participation
- Debating the barriers to lived experience research

Reflective question

As you read this chapter, we suggest you reflect on the following: How can you meaningfully include PWLE in your research project?

The historical context

The concept of involvement of PWLE in health and social care research in the UK is deeply rooted within the history of New Social Movements that emerged in the late 20th century (Barnes and Cotterell, 2011). New Social Movements led by communities with lived experience advocated for civil rights and social change. This included movements such as feminism, anti-racism, lesbian and gay and disability activism amongst others. As part of their political mobilisation, marginalised communities challenged the predominant ideology of the time that professionals knew best (Barnes and Cotterell, 2011). Activists drew attention to the potential ways in which traditional academic-led approaches to research oppressed and marginalised groups of people and led to research findings that were disconnected from the lived experience of these communities.

For example, disability activists argued that research led by non-disabled researchers justified segregation and the denial of human rights (Oliver, 1990). Moreover, since the 1960s, feminists have campaigned against gender biases within healthcare research.

Historically, for example, research has been conducted on cisgender men and the results generalised to the rest of the population. This has led to delays in treatment and ineffective or harmful interventions to other groups (Merone et al, 2022). Instead, the activists of New Social Movements argued that both research and health and social care services should be more accountable to the people whom they are supposed to serve (Barnes and Cotterell, 2011); a concept best exemplified through the rallying call of the disability rights movement – 'Nothing about us without us' (Charlton, 1998). Hence, this increased the call for PWLE to be more fully involved in health and social care research.

With the election of the New Labour Government in 1997, the need to involve 'service users' within both policy development and research became more mainstream (Cowden and Singh, 2007). There is now an expectation that health and social care research design will be informed by 'patient and public involvement' (PPI) – 'an active partnership between patients and/or members of the public and researchers' distinct from research participation (NIHR, 2021a). An important principle was founded – research should be conducted in a collaborative way with contributions from PWLE.

A radical model of democratic citizenship to compliant consumers

Whilst the importance of involving PWLE has been embedded within policy and legislation since the turn of the millennium, this co-occurred with the ongoing privatisation of the welfare state in accordance with a neoliberal policy agenda (Cowden and Singh, 2007). Disability activists have argued that this context led to their originally transformative demands being diluted, from people with lived experience making decisions based on a radical model of democratic citizenship; to compliant consumers whose voices are performatively co-opted to validate a predetermined conservative agenda (Madden and Speed, 2017). Cowden and Singh (2007, p 9) argue:

> the crucial question here is the issue of power, yet without a context in which this can be addressed the voice of the User becomes a fetish – something which can be held up as a representative of authenticity and truth, but which at the same time has no real influence over decision making.

Therefore, if researchers are not transparent about the way that power will be shared with PWLE, involvement can be tokenistic and even harmful.

Superficial involvement can have a negative impact on PWLE (especially those from marginalised communities) through promoting feelings of disappointment, isolation, and low self-worth (Staniszewska et al, 2011). It is therefore a key principle within any project to be clear about the role of people with lived experience, the level of power they will hold over decision making, and why this decision has been made. This will be an important principle to uphold in each research project, as the involvement of PWLE and the power they hold will vary depending on the project's nature and the needs of the PWLE. The following model of engagement and participation will be a useful one to consider when you plan your research project.

Models of engagement and participation

The ladder of co-production (Figure 8.1) is commonly used in research to depict the relationship, and power dynamics shared, between professionals and PWLE – moving from no involvement or power held by PWLE to fully sharing power and decision making on service user and carer-led projects.

- *Doing to*: this mirrors traditional approaches to research where the researcher holds all the power and makes all decisions. PWLE are not involved in the design, delivery, or dissemination of the research.
- *Doing for*: PWLE have limited involvement in ways that are defined by researchers or professionals. For example, they may be invited to share their views after a proposal has been made or informed about a change that will happen. PWLE are invited to share their views, but it is ultimately the decision of professionals as to how those views inform decision making. At this stage, PWLE do not hold any power over decision making.
- *Doing with*: At the top of the ladder, power is shared with PWLE. Co-design involves valuing, debating, and acting on the views of people with lived experience. Within a co-produced project, PWLE are co-researchers within a project or may lead research with support from professionals (Slay and Penny, 2014).

The ladder of co-production has been critiqued for depicting a simplistic hierarchy of participation, which has led to the development of other models; for example, the

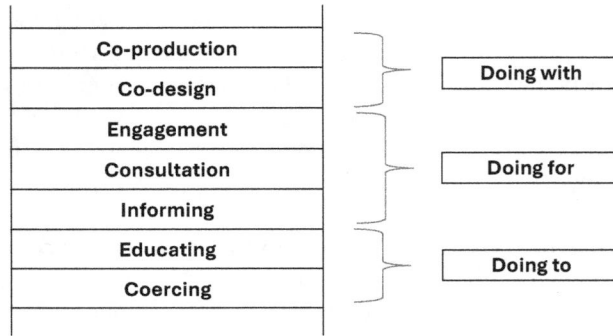

Co-production		
Co-design	}	Doing with
Engagement		
Consultation	}	Doing for
Informing		
Educating	}	Doing to
Coercing		

Figure 8.1 The ladder of co-production

participatory model by Aldridge (2014). Whilst all research should move away from considering service users or participants as passive objects, the participatory model that is chosen should be decided based on the needs and context of the community or group concerned and the role of, and power held by, participants clearly defined (Aldridge, 2014). For example, some people with learning difficulties may find it harder to understand complex theories and complete administration associated with accessing research funding, without support. Therefore, a fully participant-led approach may not always be appropriate or possible (Walmsley and Johnson, 2003). Again, the principle of what is most appropriate for the research project and the PWLE is fundamental. This concept is outlined in the following case study.

Case study

The University of Worcester's PWLE, known as IMPACT, is made up of approximately 35 service users and carers from wide-ranging backgrounds. The group was initially developed in 2008 and supports a diverse range of professional courses in areas of recruitment and selection, teaching and learning, assessment, and research.

The research by Rooney et al (2019) is an example of 'doing with' the IMPACT group (Figure 8.1). This research study sought to gain views from academic members of staff about their experiences of working with PWLE. The idea originated from an IMPACT group meeting with the academic member of staff supporting the PWLE co-researchers in the research design, analysis of findings, and the writing up of the research. PWLE co-researchers conducted semi-structured interviews with staff members. This example showed how each researcher could work together and bring their expertise to the research project. The idea for the research project was led by PWLE and consequently a more inclusive stance with more equal roles between the researchers was achieved.

Benefits of involving people with lived experience

In addition to moral and ethical benefits, there are many instrumental benefits of including PWLE in a research project. One example is the benefits of shared experience and 'insider' knowledge. PWLE may be able to better understand the experiences of research participants due to their shared experience. According to Nind and Vinha (2014), these shared experiences can inform the design of research, so it is more accessible for participants. They argue that involvement means research can reach communities that may be labelled as hard to access or underserved. Moreover, PWLE involvement in research may be considered more authentic to those in the role of respondents, by building on insider cultural knowledge (Nind and Vinha, 2014). It is therefore important in your research design to consider what is the most meaningful way to involve PWLE. The following student reflection offers an example of 'Doing for' (Figure 8.1) and highlights some of the benefits of drawing on the personal experience of a PWLE.

Student voice

At my university, we had a PWLE group. It is important we listen to the person who has lived experience, as we will never truly understand how it feels if we have never experienced it ourselves. As students, when we interacted with the PWLE group, we would gain feedback from them to tell us what worked well and what we needed to improve on before we commenced our work placements.

During my final year, I completed an empirical dissertation. This involved interviewing PWLE. My dissertation was based on the support given to families who have been affected by dementia. I met a PWLE group member who had experience caring for her mother who was diagnosed with dementia. I learned from this member, and she helped me create my questions for my interviews. Meeting with the IMPACT member made me recognise some of the language I use could affect the relationship I build with my interviewees. E.G. acknowledging the individual's names and the person with dementia rather than using "your mum or partner". This is something I had not thought about before. She was able to advise me on how to talk about the sensitive subject with those affected by dementia. I conducted semi-structured interviews with family carers. I interviewed families who were caring for their mothers/partners who were diagnosed with dementia. I thought it was important to value the PWLE if I was going to be talking about their area of expertise. As students, we have some basic knowledge, but the rest of our learning comes from the PWLE. If students are taught how important it is to work with PWLE from the beginning of their social work journey this can develop good working practices to continue post-qualification.

PWLE have said that involvement in research can enable them to develop new and existing skills, confidence, and acquire knowledge about the topics being studied from a researcher perspective. This can develop a renewed understanding of their own experience and therefore ethical considerations will need to be addressed in relation to providing support to PWLE as these new insights are realised (Diaz-Garolera et al, 2022; Puyalto et al, 2016). For some people, their interests, confidence, and skill base allow them initially to contribute in the 'Doing for' stage (Figure 8.1). This, however, provides a platform to facilitate knowledge, skills, and confidence to progress further in their research involvement. The model stage that PWLE engages with, therefore, must be determined by the needs of the PWLE alongside the research project's demands.

A further benefit to PWLE involvement in the research process relates to the concepts of PWLE feeling valued. PWLE who have been involved in research projects have highlighted significant benefits associated with feeling socially valued and developing their social networks (Diaz-Garolera et al, 2022; John et al, 2018; Nind and Vinha,

2014; Tilly, 2015). Whilst this may not be a research aim or objective, the moral and ethical advantages of such an outcome cannot be underestimated. The following student reflection shows how the aim of PWLE involvement was to increase authenticity and validity to the research project. However, there were other unintended benefits for society.

Student voice

When engaging in a research project before my final year at university, I strongly believed that without the voice of the expert by experience, findings may be inauthentic, and ethically to consider proceeding without such specialist perspectives seemed questionable, even if permissible. The research team identified personally with the subject matter, which helped participants relax and communicate comfortably. Semi-structured interview questions in the focus group provided space for exploring thoughts, opinions, and perspectives, and encouraged participants to verbalise the crucial issues that were at the heart of what mattered to them, including how services could better support them, what was helpful and, of equal importance, what was unhelpful.

Participants in the project later reported a growing sense of confidence in their knowledge and ability to challenge others around the subject, whilst one participant is now committed to a change in direction regarding her work, valuing her own voice to begin helping and supporting others going through what she herself is going through. Participating in research not only helped her to better understand her own experiences in the context of others, but also became a catalyst for commencing a journey of exploration for contributing to the education and championing of others, whilst bringing a greater awareness into the wider society in new and unique ways.

How should we consider experiential knowledge?

Some narratives of involvement can represent the knowledge constructed by PWLE as a singular 'service user voice' representing epistemic authority (Cowden and Singh, 2007). What this often means is that one person is given expert status in the belief they are the voice for a whole group of people (Trinkaus Zagzebski, 2012). In reality, PWLE often disagree between themselves (Brady et al, 2011), emphasise the complexity of their identities, and therefore reject claims that they represent their entire community (Beresford and Branfield, 2011). The term intersectionality was defined to refer to the intersection of oppressive systems that create a unique experience for people with multiple, marginalised identities. These experiences cannot be understood through the consideration of oppressive systems separately (Crenshaw, 1991). Therefore, as researchers, we need to be aware of intersectional experiences and recognise the diversity within, and between, communities and groups.

Feminist researchers have rejected the concept of a singular objective truth and instead argue that individual experiences are given meaning through engaging with cultural and community contexts. This gives rise to multiple, partial, situated knowledge (Anderson, 2014). Therefore, we should critically engage with both academic and experiential knowledge and treat neither as total, as no one person nor group can view the whole of a situation. Consequently, as you undertake a research project, it is important to consider both academic and experiential knowledge and recognise that results may not be able to be generalised to whole groups and communities.

Critiques of PWLE involvement in research

Research by Rooney et al (2019) presents some challenges of collaborative research faced by the researcher. This includes institutional, organisational, and personal challenges to the researcher:

- *institutional barriers* include bureaucracy, workload, and not being able to access PWLE easily.
- *organisational barriers* include finding additional time and energy to include PWLE in the research project and needing the PWLE to meet stringent timescales.
- *personal barriers* include perceived poor communication, for example PWLE having to decline a meeting at short notice due to ill-health (Rooney et al, 2019)

Institutional barriers include the cost of research. Budgetary constraints imposed by funding bodies can be a challenge for researchers to involve PWLE in research. Likewise, meeting the support needs of PWLE co-researchers can be expensive and time-consuming – for example, transportation costs, fluctuating health conditions or personal circumstances, and support with communication needs. Meeting these needs can be challenging for both the researcher and the PWLE involved in research (Kramer et al, 2011; Burke et al, 2015; Di Lorito et al, 2018; John et al, 2018). Meeting the support needs of service users engaged in a project takes time and resources, and these should be considered from the beginning of a project so these can be fully considered and, if needed, costed within the research budget at the application stage. Practical ways to meet the support needs of service users engaging in research can include providing interpreters, providing information in accessible or Easy Read formats, arranging meetings at times that suit individuals, enabling individuals to have support for their engagement, and providing flexibility in how individuals engage with the research. Often student researchers need to find a balance between meaningfully involving PWLE and the constraints of working without a budget. Sharing these constraints openly with PWLE can lead to a supportive environment, with PWLE knowing the expectations of their involvement. However, if we are to meaningfully address power relations that remain embedded in the 'politics of knowledge production' (Levac et al, 2019) it is important that these constraints be considered at the research design stage.

Traditionally, the body of power lies with the academic during research. Academics, therefore, need to be aware and abandon the idea of exclusionism in research, and acknowledge that PWLE involvement plays an active role and contribute to research in a practical way (Stevenson, 2014; Di Lorito et al, 2018; Levac et al, 2019). This means the role of the PWLE in the research must be clearly explained to the PWLE to ensure the integrity of data analysis (O'Brien et al, 2014). Training for PWLE can help mitigate the power differential between professionals and PWLE involved in research, particularly in co-produced research involving co-researchers. Training can focus on what research is and the skills required to conduct it. This can also have additional benefits for PWLE such as developing leadership and self-advocacy skills (van Heumen et al, 2024). Although involving PWLE in research can be beneficial, it is imperative to advocate for PWLE involved in research to be fully involved and informed of the 'now what,' in terms of dissemination after they have shared their experiences for a research topic with you (Di Lorito et al, 2018).

Personal barriers to active, collaborative involvement of PWLE include communication. For example, negotiating the language of research can be a potential challenge, as research terms are demystified into clear and concise content and contexts (O'Brien et al, 2014). Moreover, ensuring active engagement of PWLE can be challenging due to the reasons outlined in relation to institutionalised challenges (John et al, 2018). The following case study provides some solutions to address these barriers.

Case study

To overcome some of these organisational and institutional barriers the IMPACT group at the University of Worcester has an allocated facilitator and administrator. This allows for regular communication to take place between group members, academic staff members, and student researchers. IMPACT members have been part of staff training and staff meetings and have an annual IMPACT on Tour event to meet informally with academic staff. Each subject area must set aside a budget for PWLE involvement at the start of each academic year, which allows academic staff to plan their year with PWLE involvement and consultation in mind. To review progress, IMPACT members take part in staff/student liaison committees and an annual report is prepared for senior managers. These strategies support communication and the status of PWLE at the university and the sharing of expertise across course teams. This organisational structure also allows staff to better support student researchers who wish to involve PWLE in their research.

IMPACT members are given annual research training to be active members of research dialogues. This has led to co-produced or 'participant-led' projects (Aldridge, 2014) such as the example of Duddington et al (2023).

Involving PWLE as part of a co-designed or co-produced project is also a skill, and researchers need to consider their own potential learning needs. Researchers need to develop an awareness of the power dynamics inherent in interactions with PWLE and develop a reflective, and reflexive, approach to how they can empower and enable PWLE to share power and make decisions (Di Lorito et al, 2018; Levac et al, 2019; Stevenson, 2014). Adoption of the following principles can support researchers:

Sharing of power and understanding	Including all perspectives and skills	Building and maintaining relationships
Everyone is of equal importance	Working together	Decisions are jointly owned

(NIHR, 2021b)

Practical ways that researchers can enable these principles and promote their skills in co-production can include:

- Establishing ground rules and ways of working at the start of a project and regularly reviewing these to ensure they are working for everyone.
- Continually reflecting on their own use of power through keeping a reflective diary or in discussion with supervisors.
- Evaluating their approach in partnership with PWLE and giving opportunities for feedback (NIHR, 2021b).

Impact and dissemination

PWLE are often motivated to collaborate on research projects and policy development through a desire for social change and to improve circumstances for individuals or their communities. PWLE has critiqued traditional research for extracting information from a community and presenting it to academic audiences, divorced from its original values and context and having little benefit for the original respondents (Gaudry, 2011). Participatory approaches to research often acknowledge their accountability and responsibility to people with lived experience in the impact and dissemination of research (Walmsley et al, 2018). This can involve considering how to disseminate research outside of academic journals, for example sharing dissertation research within teams in the workplace and at available conferences.

Conclusion

This chapter has reflected the contemporary context of the involvement of PWLE in research. The contemporary agenda in health and social care research is now enshrined in the language of co-production, and PPI. We would argue this has been a much-welcomed move towards research with, rather than on, PWLE who have shared their experiences as part of a research study. The chapter has highlighted the benefits of involving PWLE in your research and offered examples from both a PWLE group and student researchers. Whilst there are challenges to involving PWLE in your research process, this chapter has outlined how, with careful planning, training, and value for the voices of PWLE, these can be addressed and the outcome potentially beneficial in areas you had not originally intended. We would suggest that the unique perspective offered by PWLE enhances research being undertaken and, moreover, has important moral and ethical implications for your research.

Reflective questions

1. How can people with lived experience be involved in your research?
2. How can you mitigate power dynamics when involving people with lived experience in your research?
3. What challenges do you anticipate when involving people with lived experience in your research and how might you manage these?

References

Aldridge, J (2014) *Participatory Research: Working with Vulnerable Groups in Research and Practice*. London: Sage Publications.

Anderson, E (2014) Feminist epistemology and philosophy of science. *Stanford Encyclopedia of Philosophy Online*. Available at: https://plato.stanford.edu/entries/feminism-epistemology/ (accessed 17 September 2014).

Barnes, M and Cotterell, P (2011) Introduction from margin to mainstream. In: Barnes, M and Cotterell, P (eds) *Critical Perspectives on User Involvement*. Bristol: Policy Press, pp xv–xxvii.

Beresford, P and Branfield, F (2011) Building solidarity, ensuring diversity: lessons from service users' and disabled people's movements. In: Barnes, M and Cotterell, P (eds) *Critical Perspectives on User Involvement*. Bristol: Policy Press, pp 33–46.

Bigby, C Frawley, P and Ramcharan, P (2014) Conceptualizing inclusive research with people with intellectual disability. *Journal of Applied Research in Intellectual Disabilities*, 27(1): 3–12

Brady, G Brown, G and Wilson, C (2011) Young mothers' experiential knowledge and the research process. in Barnes, M and Cotterell, P (eds) *Critical Perspectives on User Involvement*. Bristol: Policy Press, pp 149–258.

Burke, DA Koot, HM and Begeer, S (2015) Seen but not heard: school-based professionals' oversight of autism in children from ethnic minority groups'. *Research in Autism Spectrum Disorders*, 9: 112–120.

Charlton, J (1998) *Nothing About Us Without Us: Disability Oppression and Empowerment*. Oakland, CA California: Scholarship Online.

Cowden, S and Singh, G (2007) The "user": friend, foe or fetish? A critical exploration of user involvement in health and social care. *Critical Social Policy*, 27(1): 5–23

Crenshaw, K (1991) *Mapping the Margins: Intersectionality, Identity Politics, and Violence against Women of Color*. Stanford: Stanford Law Review.

Di Lorito, C et al (2018) Co-research with adults with intellectual disability: a systematic review. *Journal of Applied Research in Intellectual Disabilities*, 669–686.

Diaz-Garolera, G et al. (2022) Learnings and benefits from co-researching: views of advisors with intellectual disabilities. *Disabilities*, 2(3): 516–528. Available at: https://doi.org/10.3390/disabilities2030037

Duddington, A Gowar, D and Wall, K (2023) "Nothing about us without us": the voices of people with lived experience in practice education and post-qualifying social work. *British Journal of Social Work*, 53(3): 1766–1774.

Gaudry, AJP (2011) Insurgent research. *Wicazo Sa Review*, 26(1): 113. Available at: https://doi.org/10.5749/wicazosareview.26.1.0113

John, BS et al (2018) Reflections from co-researchers with intellectual disability: benefits to inclusion in a research study team. *Intellectual and Developmental Disabilities*, 56(4): 251–262.

Kramer, JM et al (2011) Following through to the end: the use of inclusive strategies to analyse and interpret data in participatory action research with individuals with intellectual disabilities. *Journal of Applied Research in Intellectual Disabilities*, 24(3): 263–273.

Levac, L et al (2019) A scoping review: the utility of participatory research approaches in psychology. *Journal of Community Psychology*, 47(8): 1865–1892.

Madden, M and Speed, E (2017) Beware zombies and unicorns: toward critical patient and public involvement in health research in a neoliberal context. *Frontiers in Sociology*, 2.

Merone, L et al (2022) Sex inequalities in medical research: a systematic scoping review of the literature. *Women's Health Reports*, 3(1): 49–59.

NIHR (2021a) *Briefing Notes for Researchers – Public Involvement in NHS, Health and Social Care Research*. Available at: www.nihr.ac.uk/documents/briefing-notes-for-researchers-public-involvement-in-nhs-health-and-social-care-research/27371#briefing-note-two-what-is-public-involvement-in-research (accessed 8 July 2024).

NIHR (2021b) *NIHR Co-Production in Action (Number One)*. Available at: www.learningfor-involvement.org.uk/content/resource/nihr-co-production-in-action-number-one/ (accessed 8 July 2024).

Nind, M (2017) The practical wisdom of inclusive research. *Qualitative Research*, 17(3): 278–288.

Nind, M and Vinha, H (2014) Doing research inclusively: bridges to multiple possibilities in inclusive research. *British Journal of Learning Disabilities*, 42(2): 102–109.

O'Brien, P Mcconkey, R and García-Iriarte, E (2014) Co-researching with people who have intellectual disabilities: insights from a national survey. *Journal of Applied Research in Intellectual Disabilities*, 27(1): 65–75.

Oliver, M (1990) *The Politics of Disablement*. London: Palgrave.

Puyalto, C et al (2016) Doing research together: a study on the views of advisors with intellectual disabilities and non-disabled researchers collaborating in research. *Journal of Applied Research in Intellectual Disabilities*, 29(2): 146–159.

Rooney, JM Unwin, PF and Shah, P (2019) Keeping us grounded: academic staff perceptions of service user and carer involvement in health and social work training. *Journal of Further and Higher Education*, 43(7): 929–941.

Slay, J and Penny, J (2014) *Commissioning for Outcomes and Co-Production: A Practical Guide for Local Authorities. London: New Economics Foundation.* Available at: https://neweconomics.org/2014/06/commissioning-outcomes-co-production/ (accessed 8 July 2024).

Staniszewska, S Mockford, C Gibson, A Herron-Marx, S and Johnson, R (2011) Moving forward: understanding the negative experiences and impacts of patient and public involvement in health service planning, development and evaluation. In: Barnes, M (ed) *Critical Perspectives on User Involvement*. Bristol: Policy Press, pp 129–141.

Stevenson, M (2014) Participatory data analysis alongside co-researchers who have down syndrome. *Journal of Applied Research in Intellectual Disabilities*, 27(1): 23–33.

Tilly, L (2015) Being researchers for the first time: reflections on the development of an inclusive research group. *British Journal of Learning Disabilities*, 43(2): 121–127. Available at: https://doi.org/10.1111/bld.12132

Trinkaus Zagzebski, L (2012) *Epistemic Authority – A Theory of Trust, Authority and Autonomy and Belief*. Oxford: Oxford University Press.

van Heumen, L Krueger, C and Mihaila, I (2024) The development of a co-researcher training with and for people with intellectual and developmental disabilities. *Journal of Applied Research in Intellectual Disabilities*, 37(3).

Walmsley, J and Johnson, K (2003) *Inclusive Research with People with Learning Disabilities: Past, Present and Futures*. London: Jessica Kingsley Publishers.

Walmsley, J Strnadová, I and Johnson, K (2018) The added value of inclusive research. *Journal of Applied Research with Intellectual Disability*, 31(5): 751–759.

CHAPTER 9

A secondary approach to research

Rachel Searcey and Leanne Skanta-Reading

Introduction

If you are reading this, then you are interested in health and social care research! Perhaps you are curious and want to know the differences between primary and secondary qualitative research, or you may already be in the initial query phase and wondering whether to adopt a primary or secondary approach. Whatever the reason, this chapter will give a brief overview of primary qualitative research before exploring qualitative secondary research (QSR) that equally shapes practice through the generation of new knowledge. The aims of this chapter are to raise awareness of QSR, to dispel some of the myths associated with it and to show how it is equal in value to qualitative primary research. Across this chapter, examples of how to conduct QSR will be shared from a range of health and social care secondary studies.

Chapter concepts

- Raise awareness of secondary research
- Understand the meaning of data
- Basic steps to taking a secondary approach to research
- Explore four approaches for future secondary research projects

The two research approaches

Qualitative social research systematically collects and analyses data to learn and understand more about individuals and society (Moule, 2021). The research can be influenced by personal or academic interests, fields of employment or the everyday experiences of 'what we see, hear and feel' (Largan and Morris, 2019, p 15). Whatever the line of inquiry, the research journey begins with choosing the 'best' approach to meet the study's aim (Bell and Waters, 2018).

The tendency is to adopt a primary approach by collecting new data in the pursuant of 'new' knowledge (Moule, 2021). However, researchers do have a choice: to directly

DOI: 10.4324/9781041056782-12

recruit participants using a primary research framework or search for existing data by following the steps of secondary research (Hox and Boeije, 2005). Whatever the approach, May and Perry (2022, p 2) state that all inquiries involve 'innovative thinking and meticulous attention to the details of data gathering'. Hence, the key point is that both primary and secondary qualitative research advance knowledge.

A primary method

As stated earlier, qualitative research is defined as the systematic gathering and analysis of data in response to a specific issue or problem (May and Perry, 2022). For a primary inquiry the researcher is responsible for 'choosing' the most appropriate method to collect the data in preparation for analysis (Clark et al, 2021). Yet, this is not a simple and straightforward process, 'researchers need to understand the different research methods available and learn how to apply them' (Asenahabi, 2019, p 77). For example, providing participants with diaries to record their daily experiences and behaviours captures personal insights, emotions and thoughts, or photo/object elicitation (as a visual stimulus) uncovers emotions from memory during interviews (Silverman, 2022).

Given the flexibility of qualitative research, there is no set rule for the choice of method, but this does not mean that any can be applied. Instead, the researcher needs to critically assess how the chosen method will answer the research question as each yields different data (Busetto et al, 2020). Next are three examples of the most commonly used in primary research:

- Observations: generally adopted if the inquiry seeks to better understand societal social interactions and behaviours from a health and social care perspective.
- Focus groups: if the research seeks to identify or examine similarities and/or differences from a group of individuals who share a common interest, concern, characteristic or experience.
- Interviews: to capture individual thoughts, experiences, feelings and opinions applied to individuals or groups.

(Clark et al, 2021)

In addition to *choosing* the *best* approach to collect the data, researchers also need to consider how many participants are needed for the study along with the recruitment strategy and the data analysis method. Thus, while the overarching aim of health and social care primary research is to explore or interrogate the lived experience and perceptions of the social world from as many different viewpoints as possible, it is time-consuming (Hughes and Tarrant, 2020), and requires considerable time for reflection (Hox and Boeije, 2005), preparation and sometimes training – especially if it is your first primary study (Moule, 2021). However, what is rarely considered, especially for first-time researchers, is how the data from a primary study can be utilised for a later secondary study (Largan and Morris, 2019).

The utility of a secondary research approach

The aim of any qualitative study is to capture the lived experience, behaviours, emotions and meanings attached to an individual's perspective of the social world.

To answer these specific aspects of social life, it is often perceived that one must search for new knowledge by engaging in primary research. Yet, a rarely discussed and sometimes underestimated alternative exists – secondary research. With this being said, QSR is not easier than primary research; it equally requires a robust approach in addition to a reflexive and critical mind-set (Largan and Morris, 2019). The purpose in this section is to consider the benefits of adopting a QSR approach and evidence the contribution of 'new' knowledge across the health and social care field. Heaton defines QSR as:

> A research methodology in which preexisting data are used to investigate new questions or to verify the findings of previous work. It is not to be confused with systematic reviews, literature reviews, and analysis of qualitative research, which generally involve going back over the reported findings of previous studies but not back to the original data sets, to review the state of knowledge on a given topic.
>
> (2019, p 3)

While Heaton (2019) offers an insight into QSR, she rejects the idea of consolidating findings from various sources to generate new knowledge. Furthermore, Heaton (2019) fails to acknowledge one of the core principles of research – reflection – which Hox and Boeije (2005) claim is critical to any research study including primary. However, Largan and Morris (2019) offer an alternative view. They argue that QSR is useful for:

- updating primary findings from a range of sources including published material, such as journal articles and reports for a contemporary view
- consolidating knowledge from multiple sources to create new knowledge
- revealing new insights from the primary study beyond the remit from the original study

Largan and Morris claim QSR is instead a 'reinterpretation, recontextualization, reworking or repurposing' (2019, p 13) of <u>any</u> primary data to reveal new sights. However, the dilemma presented for researchers is what actually counts as data for a secondary study. While Heaton (2019) and Moore (2007) argue against the use of journal articles claiming they lack the necessary documentary evidence to analyse experiences, Largan and Morris (2019, p 20) take a more open approach: 'we encourage you to consider documents not just as inert things, as <u>all</u> documents have a purpose and function for secondary research'. Thus, data in this sense includes journal articles, public sources (such as government and organisation reports) and data base sets (such as the UK Data Service), in addition to the original primary documentary evidence of interview transcripts, focus group reports and observation field notes/diaries. But, the researcher needs to be mindful of their over-reliance on 'published data' which could lead to descriptive findings due to the lack of direct quotes and experiences from the original primary transcripts. Wickham (2019) claims, this *waters down* the original emotive expression of feelings. While this is an important aspect to consider, one must keep in mind that all research is vulnerable to descriptive data, whether primary or secondary.

> **Reflective question**
>
> Reflect on your own understanding of research, do you consider secondary research as important as primary?

Approaching a qualitative secondary study

As discussed, the functionality of QSR is to extract and analyse existing primary or secondary data to extend knowledge and practice from various sources. The opportunities of conducting this form of research include contextualising a richer understanding from a primary study (Aveyard, 2019), exposing a different perspective (Beck, 2019), revealing new insights (Corti and Bishop, 2005) or extending the identified social phenomenon, from previous primary studies (Heaton, 2019).

QSR is integral to health and social practice and is beginning to increase in popularity (Sherif, 2018). With this initial growth, a standardised approach to document the research method is urgently needed to further promote the utility of QSR; otherwise, it will continue to remain methodically inferior to primary, and at worst viewed as a mere *literary* review of existing knowledge as opposed to the generation of new knowledge. While QSR would not exist without primary research, it is not inferior to and can be an equally exciting journey for any researcher, including students and first-time researchers.

> Among qualitative researchers, there has been a research culture that actively encourages new researchers or students in the social sciences to conduct [secondary] analysis of data collected by other researchers. Students can learn many fundamental aspects of qualitative research, and the theoretical and methodological strategies that helped to create these well-known datasets, while also gaining first-hand experience of critically re-examining original source material.
>
> (Corti and Bishop, 2005, p 9)

What Corti and Bishop (2005) show is how first-time researchers can develop research skills and be a welcomed introduction to the research field. However, as discussed, it is difficult to identify secondary research as a method (Moore, 2007). It is this particular aspect of 'researcher openness' that restricts exposure as an alternative method. As Tate and Happ (2018) note, all forms of research are important, yet it is difficult for researchers to clearly identify the mode of inquiry. Nevertheless, major funding bodies such as the Economic and Social Research Council (ESRC) now require researchers to record the chosen method in a concerted effort to advance and promote the utility of QSR. Yet, secondary research remains subsidiary to primary (Heaton, 2019). As Corti and Bishop (2005, p 8) state, 'archived qualitative data exists for it to be re-used, revisited, reanalysed and compared with other data sources.'

Overall, QSR continues to provide new insights into social life, changes in practice and new theoretical perspectives just like primary research. The evidence for this can be found in the recent reviews to explore how secondary research has been used across health and social care studies, and as anticipated, primary qualitative data is being repurposed for QSR (Heaton, 2019). Thus, while secondary research takes the researcher one step away from the original data source, it does enable the researcher to shine a different lens or closer light on the issue coming from a different angle. As Heaton (2019, p 27) notes, the 'armchair, analytical expansion' transcends findings that would have otherwise remained hidden in primary data to advance practice.

For example, a study by Watters et al (2018) captured the effects of social and economic marginalisation for lone mothers using a primary approach to research. The findings resulted in practice changes for this particular group. Yet, other notable themes such as resilience and adversity arose during data analysis but exceeded the remit of the original studies. Watters et al (2018) repurposed the original primary data to examine the earlier identified themes. This recontextualisation of existing primary data revealed a deeper understanding of the lone mother's resilient factors that would have remained unknown had the secondary study not taken place.

Initiating the secondary journey

As discussed previously, while there are many reasons why researchers adopt a secondary approach, it is not as straightforward as data collection and analysis. All researchers follow a series of methodical approaches to investigate a particular topic, problem or question, depending on the field of enquiry. As a master's student with a health and social care background, the first stage was to establish the study area which began with a scoping of the existing literature to evidence the gap (Munn et al, 2022). A useful evidence-based tool used to record and organise searches was the Preferred Reporting Items for Systematic Reviews and Meta-Analyses (PRISMA) (see www.prisma-statement.org/prisma-2020-flow-diagram for detailed guidance) and the PICO method:

- **P**: what population, patient or problem did the study focus on?
- **I**: what intervention/method strategies were adopted across the study?
- **C**: how did the study compare to other literary sources?
- **O**: what was the overall outcome of the study?

Both of these frameworks supported the 'tracking' and 'storing' of data (including academic literature) and were used interchangeably.

These two steps provided a structured approach in preparation for data collection. They also highlighted the limitations, biases and different perspectives between the primary and proposed secondary research (Moule et al, 2017). As Hughes and Tarrant (2020) state, researchers need to interrogate the original studies and locate these within their own social context. Working across the data without fully understanding these steps can lead to poor analysis, and at worse, assumptions and suppositions rather than the creation of new knowledge (Perri and Bellamy, 2012).

A further helpful starting place was Corti and Bishop's (2005) secondary research framework to consider:

- the extent and availability of data to meet the research question
- data access and restriction policies
- the range of data formats – text/audio recordings
- the extent and availability of contextual documentation
- the amount of time needed to get to know data
- researcher training needs

Following the 'scoping review' and data 'interrogation', the researcher enters the data extraction phase (from the various sources such as academic journals, reports and online databases) in preparation for analysis. It is important to acknowledge that whilst the research process is a guidance, the suggested stages ensure the research is transparent and rigorous from the outset.

The four approaches to QSR

The final section of this chapter explores the four main reasons for adopting a secondary study across health and social care that could be used as a starting point for your learning journey as a student to explore your own research ideas.

1. Comparative/Assorted Analysis. The aim of this approach will enable you as students to reveal new insights that exceed the remit of the original research. A further point that you could consider is to combine datasets or findings from a range of studies across social groups to consolidate the findings. For example, Skanta-Reading (2022) combined datasets from a range of sexual health and sexual violence studies to investigate whether survivors of sexual violence were at greater risk of contracting sexually transmitted infections (STIs). To achieve this, Skanta-Reading (2022) applied the PRISMA and PICO framework to combine the data of STI research and sexual violence research from a range of primary sources in preparation for analysis. Significantly, the secondary study revealed an increase in STIs for survivors of sexual violence compared to those who had not been exposed to sexual violence. Significantly, the knowledge from this body of research would have lay hidden within the two separate areas of research (STIs and sexual violence) had this comparative study not taken place. Moreover, Skanta-Reading (2022) notes that while comparative analysis is useful for exploring such sensitive topics, the approach is equally useful for students new to the realms of research. She argues that students are constantly engaged in exploring the current literature and thus more likely to notice the gaps across research. Therefore, comparative analysis can be an introduction to research for students and first-time researchers.

2. Research design development/advancing methodology practices. You may find within your own learning journey how this approach supports the development of new and creative ways of generating data by evaluating and/or exploring the methods utilised from primary studies. The aim is to develop 'better' strategies to capture the lived experience from participants rather than relying on the traditional methods of focus groups and interviews. For example, Pimlott-Wilson (2012) explored a range of visual data collection methods adopted across primary research and identified how the depth of information to capture a child's lived experience differed. From this, she gained a greater understanding of the varying degrees of expression and language from children and young people as participants in research. She noted how children use their everyday 'play' and 'learning' objects and art as an additional form of narration and expression of their lived world, and how these everyday play methods create a relaxed environment. All of this new knowledge from the primary research supported the creation of a new visual technique using Lego to convey meaning and adding different dimensions to the modes of language.

3. Reanalysis. This form of secondary research seeks to corroborate or verify primary findings stated in previous studies. The aim of this in health and social care research is to 'check' and 'consider' new working practices. However, while reanalysis is useful to validate or question findings from primary research, researchers fail to highlight reanalysis as the applied method. For example, Heaton's (2019) systematic review of secondary research across the health and social care sector captured only one source of QSR categorised as reanalysis. Yet, this form of research can bring a new perspective, especially if alternative methods of analysis are applied which may have not been possible at the time of the research. For students new to research, this method is equally useful for similar reasons noted by Skanta-Reading earlier (see comparative analysis). Students frequently apply a critical lens from bodies of research and draw their own findings using the literature from other bodies of research to identify new pathways.

4. Supplementary analysis. For this type of study, the researcher repurposes primary data using themes that warrant additional investigation beyond the remit of the original study. While this form of research is often carried out by the same researcher, it can also be an introduction to research for students. For instance, Hiller et al's (2023) primary study investigated the longitudinal mental health impact of the care system for young people. While the research revealed a deterioration in young people's mental health as a result of the care system, the emerging theme 'access to support' was also found across the data but beyond the remit of the study. Phillips et al's (2023) secondary study repurposed Hiller et al's (2023) data through in-depth exploration of the availability and accessibility of mental health support for young people involved in the 'system'. Together, both studies revealed two significant areas of concern around a deterioration in mental health for young people involved in the care system.

The significant difference from each of the previous examples is how each researcher defined QSR as their chosen approach in follow-up publications and included their approach to data collection. An additional key point for any student considering QSR is that if we abandon the use of data as suggested by Heaton (2019), comparative/assorted analysis and methodological development (as applied by Skanta-Reading (2022) and Pimlott-Wilson (2012) may not be utilised to advance knowledge in the way that they currently are.

> **Reflective question**
>
> Of the four approaches to secondary research discussed, which could be the most effective to your field of study, and why?

Student voice
As a student following completion of my Post-Graduate Certificate in Education, I was determined to expand my knowledge and understanding of research-based practices by pursuing a master's degree. My professional career has predominantly revolved around integrated sexual health services, providing me a rich repository of clinical proficiency, team working, leadership and management skills and counselling insight.

The decision to enrol in the MSc in leadership and health care was fuelled by a keen aspiration to make meaningful contributions to the research realm. I envisioned charting new territories in clinical practices, leaving a mark through innovative research to empower vulnerable sections of society.

Despite meticulous groundwork, including book acquisitions, seminar attendance, and exhaustive topic research, my academic journey encountered unforeseen obstacles. Originally, my ambition was to conduct primary research, to add value in healthcare. Unfortunately, the stringent confines of an 11-month window for primary research posed substantial limitations. Tasks such as navigating ethical approval procedures and recruiting participants required far more time than what was available. This was initially overwhelming which led to feelings of disappointment, as for so long I had been wanting to complete primary research and feeling that I in fact did not have a choice, and my research journey had already been mapped out based on time restrictive agents which was ultimately led by making practical decisions.

Consequently, I revised my approach midway through the program, pivoting toward secondary research – a decision made purely for practical reasons. I delved into a comprehensive systematic literature review, implementing a meticulously constructed Gantt chart which I saw as an essential component to keeping me focused and methodically self-managed amidst the wealth of information.

My journey commenced with extensive mind mapping sessions aided by mind mapping techniques. Once I developed my research focus, I embarked on a thorough scoping review across diverse databases, probing for existing evidence. Employing the PRISMA and PICO method, I meticulously structured my systematic research project that while demanded effort, unfolded into a profoundly enlightening experience.

Reflecting on this transformative experience, although my initial intent was to conduct primary research, circumstantial constraints directed me toward an equally fulfilling path of exhaustive secondary research. We need to acknowledge that while primary research is invaluable, it is not the only foundation used to shape practice. Secondary research holds significant potential in research health and social care practices, by identifying gaps, building on knowledge, and synthesising perspectives. While the journey was challenging, the lessons learned and the comprehensive insights into secondary research have indelibly shaped my outlook and encouraged my determination to pursue future healthcare secondary research.

My recommendation to anyone facing research is to set realistic and achievable goals when implementing an effective time management plan. This approach was key to keeping me on target and focused. Furthermore, the constant change when conducting research can increase anxiety and stress levels. However, by maintaining perspective, being reflective and keeping in mind the bigger picture of the why, we want to contribute to the research world.

Reflective questions

1. Now thinking about your learning as a student can you explain the significance of secondary research in comparison to primary research?

2. Can you describe a research scenario in your field where a secondary research approach would be more appropriate than a primary one? How would you apply the steps and approaches discussed in this chapter to that scenario?
3. Thinking about literature reviews, after reading this chapter do you now consider these to be secondary research? What do they add to knowledge?
4. Can you identify areas of health and social care primary research of particular interest that would benefit from a secondary research inquiry? What approach would you use?

Conclusion

Secondary research plays a critical role in exploring existing data, generating new insights and confirming findings efficiently. While primary research often dominates discussions of theory-building and data generation, secondary research has grown significantly in relevance, particularly with increased access to primary data sources with the advances of technology. We have argued that secondary data analysis is just as important as primary research, given its broader scope for applying findings.

There are many advantages to secondary research, and throughout this chapter it is shown how it complements primary research by reanalysing and contextualising data and more importantly contributes to the forever changing evidence-based practices across health and social care. Equally, secondary research in health and social research is highly regarded as an approach because of the systematic method of gathering, analysing and evaluating the vast array of research that already exists across the field of health and social care.

Final thoughts before you proceed to the next chapter: the focal point of your methodology is not heavily dependent on whether you are conducting primary or secondary research, as the fundamental processes involved in both types are similar. The significance is identifying and adapting the specific methods for collecting and analysing data to suit the specific needs of your research.

References

Asenahabi, B (2019) Basics of research design: a guide to selecting appropriate research design. *International Journal of Contemporary Applied Research*, 6: 76–89.

Aveyard, H (2019) *Doing a Literature Review in Health and Social Care: A Practical Guide*. 4th Edn. London: Open University Press.

Beck, CT (2019) *Secondary Qualitative Data Analysis in the Health and Social Sciences*. 1st Edn. London: Routledge.

Bell, J and Waters, S (2018) *Doing Your Research Project: A Guide for First-Time Researchers*. 7th Edn. London: Open University Press.

Busetto L, Wick W and Gumbinger C (2020) How to use and assess qualitative research methods. *Neurological Research Practice*, 27(2).

Clark, T Foster, Sloan L and Byrman, A (2021) *Bryman's Social Research Methods*. 6th Edn. Oxford: Oxford University Press.

Corti, L and Bishop, L (2005) Strategies in teaching secondary analysis of qualitative data. *Forum, Qualitative Social Research*, 6(1): 1–23.

Heaton, J (2019) *Secondary Analysis of Qualitative Data*. London: SAGE

Hox, J and Boeije, H (2005) Data collection, primary vs. secondary. In: Kempf, L. (ed) *Encyclopàedia of Social Measurement*. Amsterdam: Elsevier Academic Press, pp 593–599.

Hiller, RM Fraser, A Denne, M Bauer, A and Halligan, SL (2023) The development of young peoples' internalising and externalising difficulties over the first three-years in the public care system. *Child Maltreatment*, 28(1): 141–151.

Hughes, K and Tarrant, A (2020) *Qualitative Secondary Analysis*. London: SAGE.

Largan, C and Morris, T (2019) *Qualitative Secondary Research: A Step-By-Step Guide*. London: SAGE

May, T and Perry, B (2022) *Social Research: Issues, Methods and Process*. 5th Edn. London: Open University Press.

Moore, N (2007) (Re)using qualitative data? *Sociological Research Online*, 12: 1–13.

Moule, P Aveyard, H and Goodman, M (2017) *Nursing Research: An Introduction*. 3rd Edn. Los Angeles: SAGE.

Moule, P (2021) *Making Sense of Research in Nursing Health and Social Care*. London: SAGE.

Munn, Z Pollock, D Khalil, H Alexander, L McInerney, P Godfrey, C Peters, M and Tricco, A (2022) What are scoping reviews? Providing a formal definition of scoping reviews as a type of evidence synthesis. *JBI Evidence Synthesis*, 20(4): 950–952.

Perri 6 and Bellamy, C (2012) *Principles of Methodology: Research Design in Social Science*. London: SAGE

Phillips, A Halligan, S Denne, M Hamilton-Giachritsis, C Macleod, J Wilkins, D and Hiller, R (2023) Secondary data analysis of social care records to examine the provision of mental health support for young people in care. *JCPP Advances*, 3(2), e12161.

Pimlott-Wilson, H (2012) Visualising children's participation in research: Lego Duplo, rainbows and clouds and moodboards. *International Journal of Social Research Methodology*, 15(2): 135–148.

Sherif, V (2018) Evaluating preexisting qualitative research data for secondary analysis. *Forum, Qualitative Social Research*, 19(2).

Silverman, D (2022) *Doing Qualitative Research*. 6th Edn. Washington, D.C: SAGE.

Skanta-Reading, L (2023) An investigation of the impact and consequences of survivors who have been exposed to sexual violence. Masters Dissertation, University of Derby.

Tate, J and Happ, M (2018) Qualitative secondary analysis: a case exemplar. *Journal of Paediatric Health Care*, 32(3): 308–312.

Watters, E Cumming, S and Caragata L (2018) The Lone Mother Resilience Project: a qualitative secondary analysis. *Forum: Qualitative Social Research*, 19(2).

Wickham, R (2019) Secondary analysis research. *Journal of Advanced Practitioner in Oncology*, 10(4): 395–400.

Demystifying research philosophies and paradigms

Mel Lindley, Sarah Henderson and Agnella Serafin

Introduction

This chapter aims to demystify research philosophies and paradigms and consider different study designs and methodologies that are relevant to you as health and/or social care students. Social science is described as the study of people: people as individuals, communities and societies. It aims to gain understanding of behaviours and relationships between individuals and with the wider external environment (Kuper, 2004) relevant to the social science researcher; however, this is not necessarily the case.

When sitting down to write this chapter, the authors felt it important to cover a range of different methodologies within this chapter to help you appreciate that whilst qualitative research is often associated with health and social care (Kuper, 2004), quantitative and even mixed methods should not be discounted, as these methodologies can provide very important data that can help us understand the implications of the behaviours and relationships between individuals.

In order to explore why different methods might be appropriate, we need to start at the beginning: research philosophy. We will then touch on what we mean by research paradigms before exploring different methodologies and different study designs and methods (aka ways of collecting data).

This chapter is not meant to cover every possible research method or even methodology, but help you understand some key methodologies and study designs that may be of relevance to you as a health and social care student.

Chapter concepts
- Research philosophies and paradigms
- Research methodologies

  - Qualitative
  - Mixed-Methods
  - Quantitative

- Types of qualitative methods

DOI: 10.4324/9781041056782-13

Research philosophies and paradigms

In Chapter 6, the importance of defining your research aims and questions have been explored. In this chapter we will look at the different methodologies and how they align to different research aims and questions. But first, let's start with some of the technical terms associated with research philosophies.

When understanding the relationship between philosophies, paradigms, methodologies and study design (method), it's important to realise that each method exists in its own right, but it is the understanding of your philosophy as a researcher on a given subject that will ultimately influence your methodology and then the identification of the best method to allow you to answer your research question. Let's break this down:

Ontology is the research philosophy associated with the identification of what is known (Teddlie and Tashakkori, 2009), whereas epistemology relates to the nature of how knowledge is created and what kinds of knowledge are possible (Ritchie and Lewis, 2003). So basically, ontology is concerned with 'what' we know, and 'how we know what we know', and epistemology is the 'how' to gather that knowledge and trust it.

In research, we also talk about research paradigms. This term relates to how members of a research community 'view' their world, and the research methodologies they choose in order to study in that field (Sloan and Quan-Haase, 2017). Ultimately, each paradigm has its own concepts and theories on how to view the world. Let's have a brief look at these paradigms so you can consider them when we go into more detail about the research methodologies themselves.

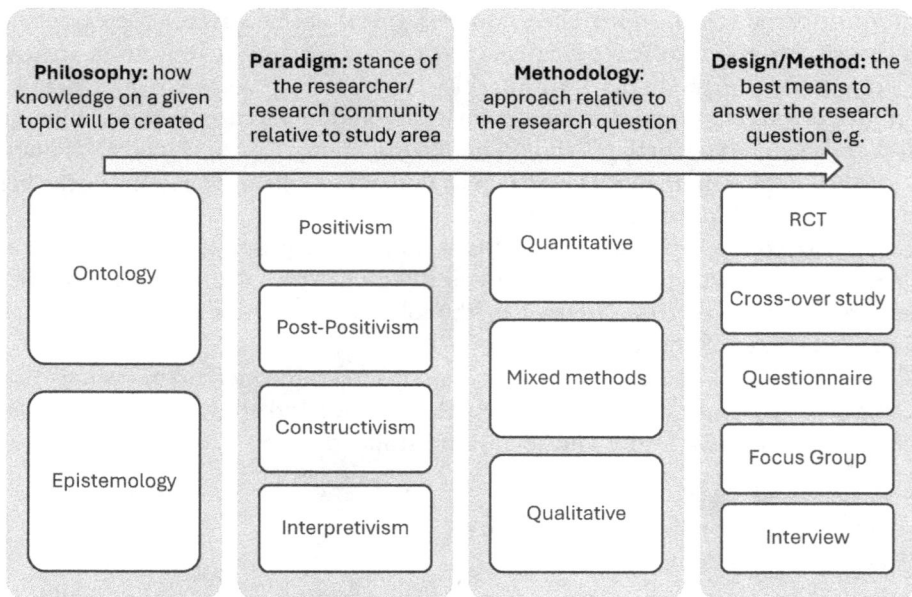

Figure 10.1 Relationship between philosophies, paradigms, methodologies and study design

Positivism

Positivism is concerned with the collection of empirical data and observations through controlled means that test hypotheses and provide identification and verification of information (Khanna, 2019). This paradigm is associated with quantitative methodologies. Positivists deem randomised controlled trials (RCTs) the 'gold standard' of research methodologies as a means of ascertaining whether an intervention works, or a theory has been proven (Beutler et al, 2014). The value of this paradigm has often been questioned, particularly by social science researchers, who consider personal, social, cultural and environmental factors as important influences on how we as individuals interpret these 'facts' and create meaning (Beutler et al, 2014). We'll come back to this assertion later in the chapter.

Post-positivism

Post-positivism asserts that whilst there is, in theory, an external reality there are multiple interpretations of that reality, based on factors such as experience, perspective and environment, each of value to those who hold the belief of that reality (Creswell and Plano Clark, 2011). The post-positivism can therefore be aligned to both quantitative and qualitative methodologies, depending on the context of the research. Post-positivist qualitative studies facilitate the gaining of insight and understanding of multiple and differing perspectives, whilst also attempting to offer clarity and sufficient agreement amongst participants that enables judgements to be formed and recommendations to be made.

Constructivism

Conversely to positivism, constructivism is concerned with how an individual constructs and makes sense of the world around them (Creswell and Plano Clark, 2011). This paradigm is also different to post-positivism as its premise is less about the different perspectives or interpretations of a given reality, and more based in the premise that each individual has their own reality.

Interpretivism

Interpretivism aligns to methodologies that provide a narrative through an inductive approach and the co-construction of data (Khanna, 2019). It also strongly integrates reflexivity by encouraging the researcher to explore their own influences on the research process through socio-psychological dialogue and reflexive elaboration. This research paradigm is of real importance in giving voice to individuals without interpretation of ideas and perspectives.

So, what does all that mean in practice, and how does this relate to research methodologies? Let's break that down and think about how you identify the most appropriate methodology for your chosen area of research.

Identifying your research methodology

In order to design and implement quality research, a balance needs to be struck between the underpinning philosophies, their respective paradigms and the most appropriate methodology for the context of the study. Ultimately, it all comes down to your research question. Chapter 6 has explored how you refine your research aims and objectives; and how you then define specific research questions. When you are defining your research question think about whether you are looking to co-construct data (interpretivism paradigm), understand an individual's reality (constructivist paradigm), wanting to gain perspectives on individuals' experiences of a given situation (post-positivism) or if you are wanting to collect empirical data (positivism), as this will lead you to different research designs.

Qualitative research methodologies

There are different types of qualitative research studies. We will briefly outline some of the types that may be of relevance. These are: phenomenological studies, ethnographic studies, grounded theory studies and action research studies.

Phenomenological studies

Phenomenological studies examine experiences through the accounts provided by the individuals involved. These are called lived experiences. The aim of phenomenological studies is to describe the meaning that experience holds for each individual. This type of research is used to study areas in which there is little knowledge (Donalek, 2004). In phenomenological research, respondents are asked to describe their experiences as they perceive them, usually through interviews. The reflexivity of the researcher is critical in phenomenological studies: they must take into account their own beliefs and feelings, as well as any pre-existing expectations; and deliberately put them aside. Only then can the researcher begin to understand the lived experience from the vantage point of the subject, seeing the experience through the eyes of the individual. Typical phenomenological research questions include the terms 'what are the experiences of ...', or 'what is it like for ...'

Ethnographic studies

Ethnographic studies involve the collection and analysis of data about cultural groups (Punch, 2013) to enable the development of cultural theories. It has been defined as the systematic process of observing, detailing, describing, documenting and analysing the actions, behaviours, lifestyles or particular patterns of a culture, or subculture. In ethnographic research, the researcher frequently immerses themselves with the people they are studying, exploring with those individuals their rituals and practices. An entire cultural group may be studied or a subgroup within a particular culture. The term culture may be used in the broad sense to describe specific groups within wider society, or groups of professionals working within specific contexts, for example. When undertaking ethnographic studies, it's important for the researcher to also interview individuals who are most knowledgeable about the culture. These people are called key informants. Additional data can be obtained through participant observation and interviews, with the data often being analysed simultaneously alongside data gathering (Punch, 2013) to enable new questions to emerge.

Grounded theory studies

Grounded theory studies are studies in which data are collected and analysed and then a theory is developed that is grounded in that data. Grounded theory research does not start with a hypothesis. Instead, it uses an inductive and a deductive approach, which means a theory emerges based on data, that is then itself tested (Morse and Richards, 2013). Grounded theory can be challenging to define and implement for the novice researcher. However, one of the benefits of grounded theory is it is flexible and, in the absence of pre-existing data, allows the research to be adapted based on emerging findings.

Action research studies

Action research is a type of qualitative research that identifies an action with the aim of improving a specified outcome, implementing that action and studying the resulting effect (Streubert and Carpenter, 2011). As the action is specific to a particular context, there is no goal of trying to generalise the findings more widely. In action research, the implementation of the potential solution occurs as an actual part of the research process, meaning that identification of problems is followed by group decisions on how to proceed. Active research must include the active participation of those who will be involved in implementing the action (Somekh, 2005). Action research does not start with a hypothesis to be tested: its purpose is to explore a particular issue, identify and implement a potential solution, and evaluate the outcome. Action research is more often conducted by practitioners as they are immersed in the context of the research itself.

Summary

As outlined, there are lots of different qualitative study designs that allow us as researchers to explore individuals, communities and societies, gaining an understanding of behaviours and relationships between individuals and with the wider external environment. We have broadly summarised these in Table 10.1. Some of the methodologies outlined here are quite complex and/or time consuming, requiring a high level of skill and reflexivity of the researcher. Therefore, many of us begin our qualitative research journey with phenomenological studies as our research questions tend to be based on theories and concepts that we have some understanding and/or experience of, but on which we want to explore the lived experiences of others. The later section 'Qualitative research methods' will therefore focus on methods most commonly associated with phenomenological studies.

Mixed methods methodologies

Mixed methods methodology synthesises both qualitative and quantitative methodologies, enabling knowledge to be constructed, and based on lived experiences (Teddlie and Tashakkori, 2009, p 89). Whilst some have argued that qualitative and quantitative paradigms are not compatible and research that combines the two is not valid (Howe, 1988), mixed methods research is now widely accepted as a robust methodology in its own right. Indeed, mixed methods research is argued to create greater meaning and insight when employed effectively (Plano Clark and Creswell, 2008).

Onwuegbuzie and Leech (2004) has argued that mixed methods research should not be rigid, but flexible, and should be designed to effectively answer the research question, combining appropriate quantitative and qualitative elements. However, mixed methods proponents have striven to create a framework and typology in order to provide a clear structure and legitimise it as a methodology in its own right; distinguishing it from quantitative and qualitative research respectively. Whilst this need for a typology and framework somewhat contradicts the premise of creativity and flexibility associated with mixed methods, it does provide guidance and commonality of language on which mixed methods researchers can base their chosen methodologies. It also enables true mixed methods research to be distinguished from multi-strand and quasi-mixed methods research.

A common pitfall in the implementation of mixed methods research is the existence of the two different paradigms within one study, but in complete isolation to one another. This is known as a monomethod multi-strand study; so defined when there is no integration between the quantitative and qualitative elements at any stage of the research process. Whilst these studies are appropriate designs in the right circumstances, it is important that two strands co-existing, albeit separately, within the same study are not conflated with genuine mixed methods.

When deciding on a mixed methods design, integration between the quantitative and the qualitative elements is key to provide opportunities for triangulation, cross analysis and meta-inference. In order to achieve this, it is important to consider the relative order and influence of each aspect of the study and the points at which they will integrate. This will help inform the stages of implementation, data collection and analysis. If integration is not apparent across the quantitative and qualitative elements, the dichotomy of the two paradigms becomes more evident.

To be classed as true mixed methods, integration of datasets either at analysis or interpretation stage is an essential component, as it is fundamental to the very purpose of supporting greater consideration of the research topic as a whole based on a culmination of outputs, perspectives and lived experiences. Sequencing of methods of data collection and/or analysis, as well as the points for integration, have led to numerous mixed methods classifications. This is not unexpected in light of the flexible and creative element of mixed methods. As can be seen in Table 10.1, there are multiple typologies with similarities across each in terms of sequencing and priorities.

Table 10.1 Outline of mixed methods typologies (adapted from Plano Clark and Ivankova, 2016, pp 112–115)

Authors	Typology	Associated Designs	Characteristics
Greene (2007)	Interactive-Independent Dimension Design Clusters	Component MM Designs: Convergence Extension	Timing: concurrent or variable Integration: at result interpretation Priority: equal or variable
		Integrated MM Designs: Iteration Blending Nesting or Embedding Mixing for Reasons of Substance or Value	Timing: concurrent, sequential or variable Integration: across all stages in a study process Priority: equal or unequal
Teddlie and Tashakkori (2009)	Five Families of Mixed Methods Design	Parallel Mixed Designs	Timing: occurs in parallel manner either simultaneously or with a time lapse Integration: at result interpretation
		Sequential Mixed Designs	Timing: sequential Integration: at connecting study phases
		Conversion Mixed Designs	Timing: concurrent or variable Integration: when transforming one type of data (e.g. qualitative) into alternative type (e.g. quantitative)
		Multilevel Mixed Designs	Timing: concurrent or sequential Integration: across multiple data levels in a study process
		Fully Integrated Mixed Designs	Timing: concurrent or sequential Integration: across all stages in a study process
Morse and Niehaus (2009)	Mixed Method Design Typology	Qualitatively Driven Mixed Method Designs Qualitatively Driven Simultaneous Qualitatively Driven Sequential	Timing: concurrent or sequential Integration: at results' interpretation or at connecting two phases Priority: qualitative

(Continued)

Table 10.1 *(Continued)*

Authors	Typology	Associated Designs	Characteristics
		Quantitatively Driven Mixed Method Designs Quantitatively Driven Simultaneous Quantitatively Driven Sequential	Timing: concurrent or sequential Integration: at results' interpretation or at connecting two phases Priority: quantitative
		Complex Mixed and Multiple Method Designs Qualitatively Driven Quantitatively Driven	Timing: concurrent or sequential Integration: at connecting multiple study phases Priority: qualitative or quantitative
Creswell and Plano Clark (2011)	Prototypes of Mixed Methods Designs	Convergent Parallel	Timing: concurrent Integration: at results' interpretation Priority: equal
		Explanatory Sequential	Timing: sequential; quantitative first Integration: at connecting two study phases Priority: quantitative
		Exploratory Sequential	Timing: sequential; qualitative first Integration: at connecting two study phases Priority: qualitative
		Embedded	Timing: concurrent or sequential Integration: included within a traditional QUANT or QUAL design Priority: unequal
		Transformative	Timing: concurrent and sequential Integration: at multiple levels as shaped by a theoretical framework Priority: variable
		Multiphase	Timing: concurrent and sequential Integration: at multiple phases within an overall programme-objective framework Priority: variable

Quantitative methodologies

While this chapter showcases the advantages and usefulness of qualitative techniques, we would be remiss to ignore the quantitative side of research methods. While your first reaction may be to think that objective, scientific and non-flexible quantitative methods may not be appropriate or helpful in the health and social care field, this section will discuss how quantitative methods should not only be considered by those in (or hoping to join) practice, but also can work extremely effectively with the qualitative techniques already discussed.

Quantitative research explores phenomena that can be objectively measured and does so through the collection of numerical data (or data that can be transformed into numbers) (Creswell, 2014). Issues such as reliability and validity need to be considered to ensure the phenomenon is accurately represented (Howitt and Cramer, 2020a; Golafshani, 2003). Quantitative research is commonly associated with the philosophical paradigm of positivism, which states that objective knowledge (facts) are gained from direct experience or observation (Cohen et al, 2011). Logical positivism takes this a step further by saying that specific testable predictions can be made from these observed facts and, through deduction, tested for veracity. This in turn leads us to the idea of the scientific, or hypothetico-deductive, method (Popper, 2005).

The hypothetico-deductive method allows us to come up with a theory about phenomena we can observe in the world. From this theory, we develop a testable hypothesis (a prediction of the phenomenon). We then test this hypothesis and evaluate the veracity of the theory we developed (Babbie, 2010).

Quantitative research is generally viewed as being systematic, generalisable, robust and scientific (Bryman, 2016). This doesn't mean that qualitative techniques are inappropriate, but merely that they are scientific and generalisable in different ways.

Application to practice

Quantitative research appears to be more popular and widely used in certain branches of social studies. It is a common technique in health-related topics, psychology, sociology and economics, but less popular in areas such as social work and anthropology (Punch, 2013). Having said this, it can effectively be used by practitioners.

Quantitative research explores trends and patterns in a population. However, since it is usually impossible to test an entire population, researchers will instead test a representative sample of the population. This means that quantitative research typically involves the use of larger sample sizes in order to avoid sampling error (Fowler, 2013). Sampling error is when the sample is not representative and is usually impossible to avoid, but certain techniques can be employed to minimise it and increase the power of the study (Howitt and Cramer, 2020b; Cochran, 1977).

These larger sample sizes and the use of standardised measures that offer easily measurable data allow clear comparisons and developments to be measured within and across samples (Fink, 2010). This clearly allows outcome results to be measured. This can be helpful in a number of contexts, such as risk assessment, which allows at-risk individuals or populations to be identified and resource allocation to be prioritised. This also allows service user outcomes to be followed over time, so interventions can be appropriately tracked and adjusted as necessary (De Vaus, 2001). Moreover, quantitative analysis can transform complex numerical data into engaging visuals, which enhances pattern identification and makes the research outcomes even more impactful. Additionally, these outcomes can be used to demonstrate value and impact to funders, stakeholders and the community. Many of them may also be using quantitative data to assess the impact within their own disciplines (Trochim and Donnelly, 2008). This allows easy integration with existing datasets, thus informing widespread practices and policies (Sharland, 2013).

Another key advantage of quantitative research is that it is objective. Qualitative research relies on the researcher's prior experience and expectations. This can be exceptionally useful, but it does mean that the researcher is viewing their data through the prism of their own bias (Denzin and Lincoln, 2011). It is impossible for research to be entirely objective; after all, why would we bother investigating something if we did not have some sort of interest in the topic? However, the increased objectivity means that the data is allowed to speak for itself without a meaning being enforced upon it by the researcher (Patton, 2002).

Quantitative research is the foundation of evidence-based practice, allowing practitioners to make sure that their knowledge is informed by systematic, robust evidence (Sackett et al, 1996). This means that interventions, treatments and teaching is based on data-driven, measurable outcomes.

Qualitative research methods
This section of the chapter outlines some methods that support qualitative methodologies. It outlines the relative benefits and limitation of each form of data collection method, as well as some practical tips.

Individual interviews
The purpose of a qualitative interview is to generate textually rich data (Kelly, 2010). It has been described as a conversation with purpose (Tilly, 2022). Qualitative interviews differ from structured interviews, which have very fixed questions and fixed choice answers, are conducted in a standardised manner and generate quantitative data (Tilly, 2022). Instead, qualitative interviews aim to gain individual participants' insights, experiences and/or perspectives. This can be done through semi-structured or unstructured interviews.

Semi-structured interviews require the researcher to develop a series of themes or topics in advance of the interview, based on the research questions. You may hear this referred to as being a 'topic guide'. If you are developing a topic guide, think about the areas you want to explore. You will need to balance how you explore the meanings and perspectives of participants with the need to gain data that enables you as the researcher to answer your research questions/objectives.

In developing your topic guide, you may wish to shape some open-ended questions for each of these areas, with some possible follow-up questions. Once you have developed this, spend some time reviewing your questions and consider whether they are potentially leading or biased to your perspective as a researcher. A significant challenge in undertaking semi-structured interviews is how, as the researcher, you ensure 'rigour' (aka good quality) without being so structured that you lose the subjectivity and richness of data generated by each participant. Key to this, but out of scope of this chapter, is the need for the researcher to demonstrate reflexivity as to their own biases, experiences and influences. This is equally true when conducting focus groups and developing questionnaires.

Focus groups

Focus groups can be an effective method in qualitative studies when a researcher wants to gain group perspectives and/or consensus, experiences of new (or established) services or an understanding of 'norms' (Barbour, 2010). They usually involve a minimum of 6 and a maximum of 12 participants taking part simultaneously in person or online (Smithson, 2008). Focus groups are extremely useful in eliciting responses to issues that do not require going into depth from individual perspectives. The group situation facilitates participants to consider matters that they may not have previously considered. This has been identified as one of the most significant advantages of focus groups as compared to other methods (Barbour, 2010). Like semi-structured interviews, the researcher will need to develop a 'topic guide' around the research objectives with open questions or statements that the participants can explore and discuss.

Questionnaires

Questionnaires and surveys can span both quantitative and qualitative methodologies. Depending on the types of questions asked, different types of data can be generated. Quantitatively speaking, there are different types of data that can be generated by a survey/questionnaire: nominal data (mutually exclusive categories, e.g. yes:no), ordinal data (ranking scales but the distance between each category is not defined, e.g. high–low), interval data (scale where the distance between the scales is defined, e.g. temperature) or ratio data (full scale with absolute zero, e.g. marks out of 100). They can also be utilised to generate qualitative data; however, designing high-quality questionnaires that enable the respondent to provide rich data requires careful consideration of language (Krosnick, 2018). Within the context of this chapter, we will not be going into detail about questionnaires or surveys, other than to encourage you, if you are thinking of using questionnaires as your method, to explore the many resources available supporting the development of quality surveys and questionnaires.

Summary

This chapter has hopefully enabled you to better understand research philosophies and paradigms, and how these, in turn, inform the research methodology for a given topic. Whilst the predominant focus of the chapter is qualitative research methodologies and methods, we hope that you now appreciate the quantitative–mixed-methods–qualitative continuum; and how each has a place in health and social care research.

Reflective questions

Which paradigm do you think phenomenological studies align to? How might the research questions of post-positivism and constructivism differ in phenomenological studies?

Think about how you could investigate an issue that you find interesting from a quantitative perspective. Or think about how you could transform something you have investigated using a qualitative technique into a quantitative project.

References

Babbie, ER (2010) *The Practice of Social Research*. 12th Edn. Wadsworth.

Barbour, R (2010) Focus groups. In: Bourgeault, I Dingwall, R and De Vries, R (eds) *The SAGE Handbook of Qualitative Methods in Health Research*. London: SAGE Publications Ltd, pp 327–352

Beutler, LE Forrester, B and Shahar, G (2014) What needs to change: moving from 'research informed' practice to 'empirically effective' practice. *Journal of Psychotherapy Integration*, 24(3): 168–177.

Bryman, A. (2016) *Social Research Methods*. 5th Edn. Oxford: Oxford University Press.

Cochran, WG (1977) *Sampling Techniques*. 3rd Edn. New York: John Wiley & Sons.

Cohen, L Manion, L and Morrison, K (2011) *Research Methods in Education*. 7th Edn. London: Routledge.

Creswell, JW (2014) *Research Design: Qualitative, Quantitative, and Mixed Methods Approaches*. 4th Edn. Los Angeles: SAGE Publications Ltd.

Creswell, JW and Plano Clark, VL (2011) *Designing and Conducting Mixed Methods Research*. 2nd Edn. Los Angeles: SAGE Publications Ltd.

De Vaus, DA (2001) *Research Design in Social Research*. London: SAGE Publications Ltd.

Denzin, NK and Lincoln, YS (Eds) (2011) *The SAGE Handbook of Qualitative Research*. 4th Edn. Los Angeles: SAGE Publications Ltd.

Donalek JG (2004) Phenomenology as a qualitative research method. *Urol Nurs*, 24(6): 516–517. PMID: 15658739.

Fink, A (2010) *Conducting Research Literature Reviews: From the Internet to Paper*. 3rd Edn. Los Angeles: SAGE Publications Ltd.

Fowler, FJ (2013) *Survey Research Methods*. 5th Edn. Los Angeles: SAGE Publications Ltd.

Golafshani, N (2003) Understanding reliability and validity in qualitative research. *The Qualitative Report*, 8(4): 597–607.

Greene, JC (2007) *Mixed Methods in Social Inquiry*. California: John Wiley & Sons.

Howe, KR (1988) Against the quantitative-qualitative incompatibility thesis or dogmas die hard. *Educational Researcher*, 17(8): 10–16.

Howitt, D and Cramer, D (2020a) *Research Methods in Psychology*. 6th Edn. Harlow: Pearson Education Limited.

Howitt, D and Cramer, D (2020b) *Understanding Statistics in Psychology with SPSS*. 8th Edn. Harlow: Pearson Education Limited.

Kelly, S (2010) Qualitative interviewing techniques and styles. In: Bourgeault, I Dingwall, R and De Vries, R (eds) *The SAGE Handbook of Qualitative Methods in Health Research*. London: SAGE Publications Ltd, pp 307–326

Khanna, P (2019) *Positivism and Realism*. Singapore: Springer.

Krosnick, JA (2018) Questionnaire design. In: Vannette, DL and Krosnick, A (eds) *The Palgrave Handbook of Survey Research*. London: Palgrave, pp 439–455.

Kuper, A (Ed) (2004) *The Social Science Encyclopaedia*. 3rd Edn. London: Routledge.

Morse, JM and Field, PA (1996) Principles of conceptualizing a qualitative project. *Nursing Research: The Application of Qualitative Approaches*. New York: Springer, pp 35–55.

Morse, JM and Niehaus, L (2009) *Mixed Method Design: Principles and Procedures*. Walnut Creek, CA: Left Coast Press.

Morse, JM and Richards, L (2013) *Qualitative Research Design. Readme First for a User's Guide to Qualitative Methods*. 3rd Edn. Los Angeles, CA: Sage.

Onwuegbuzie, AJ and Leech, NL (2004) Enhancing the interpretation of 'significant' findings: the role of mixed methods research. *The Qualitative Report*, 9(4): 770–792.

Patton, MQ (2002) *Qualitative Research and Evaluation Methods*. 3rd Edn. California: SAGE Publications Ltd.

Plano Clark, VL and Creswell, JW (2008) *The Mixed Methods Reader*. London: SAGE Publications Ltd.

Plano Clark, VL and Ivankova, NV (2016) *Mixed Methods Research: A Guide to the Field*. Los Angeles: SAGE Publications Ltd.

Popper, KR (2005) *The Logic of Scientific Discovery*. London: Routledge.

Punch, KF (2013) *Introduction to Social Research: Quantitative and Qualitative Approaches*. 3rd Edn. Los Angeles: SAGE Publications Ltd.

Ritchie, J and Lewis, J (2003) *Qualitative Research Practice—A Guide for Social Science Students and Researchers*. London, Thousand Oaks, CA: Sage Publications Ltd.

Sackett, DL Rosenberg, WM Gray, JA Haynes, RB and Richardson, WS (1996) Evidence-based medicine: what it is and what it isn't. *BMJ*, 312(7023): 71–72.

Sharland, E (2013) Where are we now? Strengths and limitations of UK social work and social care research. *Social Work and Social Sciences Review*, 16(2): 7–19.

Sloan, L and Quan-Haase, A (2017) *The SAGE Handbook of Social Media Research Methods*. London: SAGE Publications, Ltd.

Smithson, J (2008) Focus groups. In: Alasuutari, P Bickman, L and Brannen J (eds) *The SAGE Handbook of Social Research Methods*. London: SAGE Publications Ltd, pp 357–370.

Somekh, B (2005) Action Research. New York: McGraw-Hill Education (UK).

Streubert, HJ and Carpenter, DR (2011) *Qualitative Research in Nursing: Advancing the Humanistic Imperative*. Philadelphia: Wolters Kluwer.

Teddlie, C and Tashakkori, A (2009) *Foundations of Mixed Methods Research: Integrating Quantitative and Qualitative Approaches in the Social and Behavioral Sciences*. Los Angeles, CA: SAGE Publications Ltd.

Tilly, L (Ed.) (2022) *Health and Social Care Research Methods in Context: Applying Research to Practice*. Oxon, UK: Routledge, Taylor & Francis Group.

Trochim, WM and Donnelly, JP (2008) *The Research Methods Knowledge Base*. 3rd Edn. Mason, OH: Atomic Dog Publishing.

CHAPTER 11

Creative tools of research

Melanie Durowse and Var Gibson

Introduction

When thinking about undertaking research, practitioners often have a focus about what they want to find out before deciding which methodology to use. There is a huge range of methodologies, so finding one that can fit can be a challenge. For social care research, many of the methodologies can establish factual information, but may not be as effective in 'discovering the emotional reasons behind behaviour' (Richards, 2012, p 781). With that in mind, this chapter starts with a look at the political and theoretical context of social research and highlights a range of creative tools that could be used effectively, where the meaning of the responses is significant to the area of research. This will be followed by an explanation of Q sort methodology (Watts and Stenner, 2012) and our thoughts about its effectiveness as a creative tool.

Creative tools of research have been developed in response to some of the limitations of traditional methods of research. More conventional research methods often focus on quantitative data gathering, requiring a high level of responses with the researcher analysing the results. Questionnaires, for example, are a respected tool as they deliver high volume data (Robson, 2011). However, Einola and Alversson (2021) noticed when they observed people completing questionnaires that some people were confused about the question being asked, the question was not relevant to their experience, or the cultural understanding of particular words had different meanings. Where participants find the questions are not relevant to their experience, they may opt out and this has an impact on the data that can be extracted from a limited number of questionnaires returned. Additionally, with fixed answer questions or multiple-choice answers it is not possible to extract meaning beyond the question, unless there is space for free text responses. For social science research, there is generally a much higher importance to the interpretative nature of the findings, which requires the voice of the participants to be central to the process. The more creative tools allow for a wider engagement in the research process by hearing the voice of the individual through their personal interpretation, which in turn provides richer qualitative findings.

DOI: 10.4324/9781041056782-14

The social and political contexts of research

When seeking the views of individuals in social care research it is important to consider the wider factors impacting on their experience, particularly in relation to health. Over the years, the dominant healthcare model is that of the biomedical model (Wade and Halligan, 2017), which works on the basis that good health is due to the absence of ill health. However, the wider social determinants reflected in the social model of health (Rahman et al, 2024) of mental, physical, and social wellbeing may be related to an underlying health condition but are not necessarily linked to being ill. However, the social ecological model (Podgorski et al, 2021) places a higher significance on the connection between the individual, their views, and environment the individual is in. This allows for a better understanding of the lived experience and the interconnected factors that can limit or enhance the individual's life.

In more recent years there has been some acceptance that the voice of the individual should be central with the development of policies and legislation to support a more integrated approach to the wider needs of individuals that encompasses the determinants of wellbeing. In Scotland, the development of the Health and Social Care partnerships, incorporating National Health and Wellbeing Outcomes directing the effective use of resources and communities, states that 'people are able to look after and improve their own health and wellbeing' (Scottish Government, 2015). Effectively, this places the responsibility for community resources in the hands of those people who wish to develop and support a particular resource. For people with a cognitive impairment, such as dementia, their ability to arrange a service to meet their needs may be beyond their skills and capacity. Although carers could support such a development, there is significant evidence to indicate their caring role limits their ability to develop resources to support the person they care for (Greenwood et al, 2019).

At the same time, a reduction of funding for the health and social care is a direct result of austerity measures taken at a UK level. An analysis of the cuts to public sector funding noted the direct impact on health, environment, and housing services (Stuckler et al, 2017) and highlighted the importance of social supports, alongside the need for an appropriate environment. Therefore, the policies acknowledge the need for a person-centred approach and the introduction of wellbeing outcomes supports this direction, but the reduction in funding negates the development of resources.

In the context of social research, we are aware that the environment needs to be well-adapted to the individual, so that it can encourage people to join in, participate, and expand their circles of social support. As Beckett and Campbell (2015) emphasised, a social model of disability can highlight the barriers and limitations that make it less possible for people with disabilities or impairments. This is particularly relevant to accessibility for people with dementia. Foucault's Oppositional Device Theory (Vidler et al, 2014), that oppression can be fought with raised awareness, is relevant to the way policy is developed. The updated dementia strategy (Scottish Government, 2023) was developed by the National Dementia Lived Experience Panel and their knowledge led to a strategy that provided specific information about what people with dementia should expect. Dementia is an umbrella term for a deteriorating cognitive condition that affects memory, thinking skills, and physical health, and impacts on the individual and family members, many of whom take on a caring role. Although the strategy acknowledged there were areas that required further development, we wanted to explore how effective the strategy was in informing us about the reality of their experience. As dementia is a deteriorating condition, there are changes to people's abilities and skills as they progress through their dementia journey, and it was important to understand if the strategy was as relevant to people at different stages; in essence, to understand if the strategy reflected the reality of people's experience.

Creative tools of research
Generally creative tools are used to gather qualitative data using narrative and artistic methods to create knowledge, and their purpose is to develop deeper and richer understanding through the nuance of personal constructs. These tools can create new ways of knowing through drawing on the lived experience. Thorough listening to the participants' perspectives encourages a more equal balance between participant and researcher, limiting power imbalances that can occur. A number of creative tools have been discussed next, with each method focussing on gathering the individual perspective; most are not reliant on literacy skills, therefore could be more accessible to a wider range of participants.

Diaries
The use of diaries as a research tool is similar to a questionnaire, with the parameters of the information being gathered set by the researcher, but the participant can provide more depth to the information. It benefits the participant through the process of recording their data which allows for reflection and potentially encourages their understanding of themselves (Olorunfemi, 2024). Like questionnaires, diaries can be used independently of a group environment, but it has the advantage of valuing the uniqueness of each participant's experience. Diaries also have the added advantage of providing longitudinal data, in comparison to many other methods which are a viewpoint at a specific time. This is particularly relevant to health and substance use studies, where the data may change over time (Elliot, 1997). However, the self-reporting nature of diaries can lead to bias or misreporting, and it is suggested that a second form of data collection is considered (Robson, 2011).

Visual images
Using photographs is considered to be collaborative research (Winton, 2016) due to the engagement and active participation of the production of knowledge by those involved in the research. Whether it is through participants taking their own photographs, the use of photographs provided by the researcher, or participants seeking images to discuss, these methods are about participants interpreting the image. These methods allow the researcher to gain an understanding of the individual perspective on the image, and the different levels of meaning (Glaw et al, 2017). Commonly used as a research tool with young people, it is also a valuable tool to use with any age group where literacy may be an issue. The strength of these methods is the ability to understand the personal constructs of the image being presented and, importantly, the significance to the participant. Through exploring the way the image is perceived it can also be used in discussions to aid further understanding around particular issues.

Story telling

Based on narrative inquiry, story telling starts with a prompt from the researcher such as 'tell me a story about …' and the researcher continues to prompt the participant to keep the dialogue progressing. These types of stories provide information about the lived experience of the participant and elicits the significance of particular events (Haddington and Martin, 2012). This is particularly valuable for participants who feel their story is being told for them, and marginalised groups. However, children are often involved in child play activities of imagination, and their stories are considered to be a natural understanding of their world (Richards, 2012). As a research tool, the use of stories can inform us about feelings and emotions, which builds from the human need to communicate. The process of telling the story also can create a sense of belonging and reflection in helping the participant to make sense of events. To engage in storytelling as a research method, it requires the researcher to be accepting and nurturing with the personal narratives to counter the potential judgemental and stigmatising attitudes the participants have previously faced. It is also important to note that story telling is distinct from focus groups, as the participants should be afforded the opportunity to tell their whole story from their perspective, and the role of the researcher is to encourage that process, rather than leading a discussion on particular themes. However, the telling of individual stories does make this a more time-consuming form of data gathering for the researcher, but has the benefit of being able to be used with all individuals.

World café

Another creative participatory method to collect qualitative data, which encourages cross table discussion, is a world café. Small groups are seated in the style of a café with paper tablecloths. Each table is given a question to discuss and record their comments on the tablecloth. After a fixed period of time, the members disperse to other tables to discuss the same question with other participants. The participants are able to see the comments recorded on the tablecloths and build on those points or introduce new themes in response to the question. The sharing of ideas between participants draws on the lived experiences and perceptions, in a non-threatening environment. As with the other tools identified, this method also allows for constructive dialogue, which encourages participants to engage in collective understanding of the matter under discussion. The café styling is designed to encourage informal conversations, but in a structured context with the use of a question. It is important that the question is open enough to encourage a range of discussion points, and although it has some literacy requirements as people record their observations, symbols or drawings could be used. Although there are similarities with this approach and focus groups, this method does not require a facilitator to encourage discussions, and conversations evolve through building on the contribution of others (Lohr et al, 2020).

Q sort

Like the other creative tools of research, Q sort explores the different factors that inform the participants' thoughts.

Often referred to as a mixed methods approach (Robson, 2011), Q sort combines statistical data with narrative analysis and has strengths in exploring subjectivity (van

Exel and de Graaf, 2005) to gather 'socially relevant results' (Gomez, 2014, p 318) or establish perspectives (Billard, 1999), and is based on the Gestalt concept that perspective is mostly based on parts of an issue which are related to other issues (Gross, 2015). The research is conducted in two parts: participants rank a series of statements, known as the q set, and then discuss the ranking to determine the reason for the rank.

Whilst there is no requirement for q set to be based on specific theory (Watts and Stenner, 2005), it can draw from literature, personal experience, observations, or from more abstract ideas that will promote discussion. As we wanted to look at the lived experience of dementia, we developed our statements from government policy and health information. For example, the Dementia Strategy (Scottish Government, 2023) states high quality support and care includes 'recognising and respecting people's rights and values and putting people at the centre of care' (p 30). From this information, the q statement developed was: 'People with dementia are respected and valued'.

Creating the statements was a valuable learning process for me. I wanted to create statements that encouraged discussion and recognised our profession is often deficit based which informed my occupational views. So it was important that we stepped out of social care jargon, such as referring to outcomes, and explore what would make sense to the people who participated. It really made us think about our professional language and where it could be misunderstood. For example, the strategy refers to reducing stigma, but we didn't know if the participant had experienced negativity about their conditions and reworded it to ask if they thought society assumed people with dementia were senile or incapable. This way, we were able to have a discussion, rather than ask directly if they have been stigmatised. We checked the statements were appropriate for the participants with the use of an expert sampler. Our expert was knowledgeable about both the subject matter and how to communicate effectively to ensure participants were able to understand the q statement and respond to it.

The usual way for participants to rank their responses is through the use of a forced matrix or grid, such as the one in Figure 11.1.

The participants put the number of the q statement into the box under the category that matches how they feel about the statement. For example, if the participant completely agreed with q statement 1 from our research '*I have been given clear information about services for people with dementia*', they would write 1 in the box immediately below 'completely agree'.

The purpose of the matrix is to 'force' the participants to rank the q statements which helps them decide which are statements they have strong feelings about compared to other statements. The boxes have the effect of making participants reconsider the ranking of statements, which can lead to a refinement of their beliefs (Brown, 1980) and consider the differences (Watts and Stenner, 2012). These areas of difference should be part of the discussion in the second part of the research.

However, it is also possible to use a free distribution method, such as a Likert scale, where the participants are asked to rank the q statements on the same categories but are not forced to readjust their statements to fit into the available boxes. Watts and Stenner argue there are 'no major repercussions' from using this method (2012, p 78). For small scale studies, with low numbers of participants, it may be preferable to use a Likert scale.

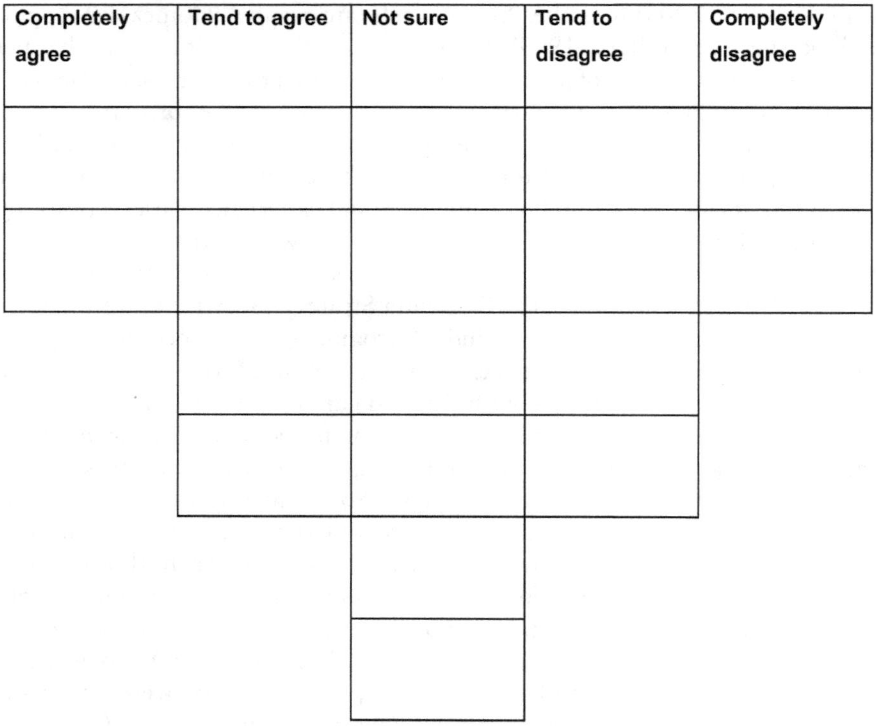

Completely agree	Tend to agree	Not sure	Tend to disagree	Completely disagree

Figure 11.1 Forced distribution score matrix

Our experience of using a forced matrix highlighted some issues that had not been considered. Dementia is characterised by an intellectual impairment and can result in difficulty retaining new information, handling complex tasks, and coping with unexpected events (Carr et al, 2000). In introducing the forced matrix, we gave a new piece of information that could be considered as a difficult task for someone with a cognitive impairment and difficulties retaining information. In asking the participant to arrange the statement in the grid, where each statement had to fit into one box, there was a level of confusion about the task. This was time consuming as we had to stay with the participants and their carers to remind them about the task and how to place the statements. People with dementia and their carers found it very challenging to fit all the statements into the boxes as there were so many 'not sure' responses.

When we discussed the position the statement had been placed in, sometimes participants would go off the subject. Although it could be a bit frustrating to lose the focus of discussion, important new information was shared which was really valuable, as it provided further context to the issues. In retrospect it would have been much easier for the participants to have used a Likert scale, but we may not have had the rich discussions that occurred while the participants were ranking the statements.

The ranking process is followed by a discussion to find out the reason the participant determined the position of the statement and establish the factors they took into account when deciding where to position the statement. The researcher's role is to encourage the participant to expand on their thoughts and experiences, to understand how they developed that particular viewpoint, and identify the factors they considered.

For example, a participant scored the statement '*I have been given clear information about services for people with dementia*' as 'not sure' and commented that at the time the information was given it was clear and understandable, but he was unable to retain the verbal information and unable to recall who had provided it so that he could ask them again.

As some of the participants encountered difficulties with the ranking process, the discussions were able to unpick their experiences which revealed inaccuracies and differences between the comments and their grid placements. This highlighted the need for a flexible approach when analysing data and the importance of involving participants to point out flaws and limitation of the method for future adaptation. Therefore, the discussion part of the research is just as crucial. It provided people with dementia and carers the opportunity to voice their views and join the scientific discourse. Despite the challenges of using the forced matrix, we gathered interesting points about how people with dementia actually felt and what they experienced. Involvement of carers helped respondents feel more open to express their views. Carers assisted in explaining what may have appeared a puzzling task for someone with a cognitive impairment. The carers were able to personalise the statements for the participants and encourage them to express their view, and was, in our opinion, crucial.

Bringing together the response to key themes is the final stage of the research, as the analysis represents the level of agreement or disagreement between the different responses, so the aim is to identify the natural groupings. Therefore, there is a need to identify similarities and differences between the scores and provide the information from the discussions to provide context to the positions.

A grid, such as Figure 11.2, records the number of statements ranked in each area, which in this case indicated there was a higher sense of agreement with statement 1, whereas statement 15 had an equal spread of views across the scoring areas.

Student voice

As a student engaging in my first significant research project, I noted that quantitative research can be very rigid and focused on data, and qualitative research can explore emotions, opinions, and ideas. By using Q sorts and adding a discussion to interpret the grid, we not only empowered and included participants into research and scientific discourse, we also actively stood up against neoliberal values (Venugopal, 2015). Our social care background made me a little sceptical when participants responded to a statement saying they had no issue using the bus. As a professional, I would ask additional questions and make sure the person actually could get on the bus, observe them at the bus stop, learn about their supports in the community, and seek collateral information from multiple sources (Dickson et al, 2023). However, as a researcher, I could not acquire this information, nor was it relevant to understanding their viewpoint. I had to record what people said and use their perceptions, which was a shift in mindset for me. By not questioning the truth and objective possibility behind statements of participants, 'I can use a bus no bother', we focused on the feelings, belief in participants' own abilities, and perception of their strengths. We enjoyed the process and focused on

Statement number	Statement	Score				
		Completely agree	Tend to agree	Not sure	Tend to disagree	Completely disagree
1	I have been given clear information about services for people with dementia	2	3	2	0	0
15	People working in services are skilled in communicating with people who have dementia	2	1	2	1	1

Figure 11.2 Analysis of scoring

exploration of people's opinions. Perhaps it may not bring as much profit as carefully presented statistics, however, it brought a benefit to the members of public, which is hard to measure, but easy for us, researchers, to see. Participants were reminded that they are the experts of their lives and abilities, and their opinions are valuable assets for research. Only people who truly experienced the environments as people with dementia, and their carers, can know how it feels to struggle within certain settings that are not well adapted and not inviting for people with a cognitive impairment. This direct lived experience is what discussions, though timely and requiring additional preparation and skills, helped us to explore. Overall, I found the process of research fascinating and learnt so much from the people we spoke to. In some cases, we weren't sure who was a carer and who was a person with dementia, but I realised that it wasn't important to identify them as their joint experience was important. Sometimes the participant strayed off topic, but even then, it gave me a real understanding of their world.

Conclusion

There is no one-size-fits-all methodology that covers all situations, but free-flowing is discussion that supports the person's view to be heard. The creative tools of research seek to hear the individual perspective and place them in the centre to share the unique knowledge they have gained through their situation. For the optimal results when working with people who have a cognitive condition, the ideal environment is quiet with researchers working at a pace suitable to the person and involving carers who help the adult to understand the statements and participate in the discussion. Knowing the right environment for the participants is key, as we found it helped to build trust and rapport. Although it was useful for our research to involve carers to support the process, it could be counterproductive when undertaking research with people who are able to express their own view without support, particularly where the participants have felt their experience has not been valued. The use of an expert in the development of the research process in Q sort is an effective way of ensuring the wording of the statements is tailored to the participant, and unambiguous. It would be useful to consider an expert in other creative methods of research to ensure the research tool will be accessible to the participants, is framed in the right language, and takes account of skill levels, cultural issues, and the ways to engage to encourage participation. Although participants may go off track and not respond to the question being asked, the information gathered is still useful. We gathered invaluable, surprising, and informative opinions from participants, improving our understanding of the issues and difficulties people with dementia and their carers face.

References

Beckett, AE and Campbell, T (2015) The social model of disability as an oppositional device. *Disability & Society*, 30(2): 270–283. www.tandfonline.com/doi/full/10.1080/09687599.2014.999912#d1e476

Billard, S (1999) How Q methodology can be democratized. *Feminism and Psychology*, 9(3): 357–366.

Brown, S (1980) *Political Subjectivity: Applications of Q Methodology in Political Science*. London: Westford.

Carr, DB Gray, S Baty, J and Morris, JC (2000) The value of informant versus individual's complaints of memory impairment in early dementia. *Neurology*, 55(11): 1724–1727. https://pubmed.ncbi.nlm.nih.gov/11113230/

Dickson, K Gala, GJ and Moseley, DD (2023) The role of decision-making capacity in gathering collateral information. *Journal of Clinical Ethics*, 34(2): 123–127. www.journals.uchicago.edu/doi/abs/10.1086/724231

Einola, K and Alversson, M (2021) Behind the numbers: questioning questionnaires. *Journal of Management Inquiry*, 30(1): 102–114.

Elliot, H (1997) The use of diaries in sociological research on health experience. *Sociological Research Online*, 2(2). www.socresonline.org.uk/2/2/7.html

Glaw, X Inder, K Kable, A and Hazleton, M (2017) Visual methodologies in qualitative research: autophotography and photo elicitation applied to mental health research. *Internation Journal of Qualitative Methods*, 16: 1–8.

Gomez, A (2014) New developments in mixed methods with vulnerable groups. *Journal of Mixed Methods Research*, 8(3).

Greenwood, N Pound, C Brearley, S and Smith, R (2019) A qualitative study of older informal carers' experiences and perceptions of their caring role. *Maturitas*, 124: 1–7.

Gross, R (2015) *Psychology: The Science of Mind and Behaviour*. London: Hodder Education.

Haddington, B and Martin, B (2012) *Universal Methods of Design: 100 Ways to Research Complex Problems, Develop Innovative Ideas, and Design Effective Solutions*. Beverley: Rockport Publishers.

Lohr, K Weinhardt, M and Sieber, S (2020) The "world café" as a participatory method for collecting qualitative data. *International Journal of Qualitative Methods*, 19: 1–15.

Olorunfemi, D (2024) Diary studies in research: more than a research method. *International Journal of Market Research*, 66(4): 410–427.

Podgorski, C Anderson, S and Parmar, J (2021) A biopsychosocial-ecological framework for family-framed dementia care. *Frontiers in Psychology*, 12: 1–15.

Rahman, R Reid, C Kloer, P Henchie, A Thomas, A and Zweiggelaar, R (2024) A systematic review of literature examining the application of a social model of health and wellbeing. *European Journal of Public Health*, 34(3): 467–472.

Richards, M (2012) Creative workshops as a qualitative research tool. *International Journal of Market Research*, 54(6): 781–789.

Robson, C (2011) *Real World Research*. Chichester: John Wiley & Sons.

Scottish Government (2015) *National Health and Wellbeing Outcomes*. Available at: www.gov.scot/binaries/content/documents/govscot/publications/advice-and-guidance/2015/02/national-health-wellbeing-outcomes-framework/documents/national-health-wellbeing-outcomes-framework-improving-planning-delivery-integrated-health-social-care-services/national-health-wellbeing-outcomes-framework-improving-planning-delivery-integrated-health-social-care-services/govscot%3Adocument/00470219.pdf (accessed 3 December 2024).

Scottish Government (2023) *Dementia in Scotland: Everyone's Story*. Available at: www.gov.scot/publications/new-dementia-strategy-scotland-everyones-story/pages/9/ (accessed 10 July 2024).

Stuckler, D Reeves, A Loopstra, R Karanikolos, M and McKee, M (2017) Austerity and health: the Impact in the UK and Europe. *European Journal of Public Health*, 27(4): 18–21. https://academic.oup.com/eurpub/article/27/suppl_4/18/4430523#113355107

van Exel, J and de Graaf, G (2005) *Q Methodology: A Sneak Preview*. Available at: https://qmethod.org/portfolio/van-exel-and-de-graaf-a-q-methodology-sneak-preview/ (accessed 24 April 2021).

Venugopal, R (2015) Neoliberalism as concept. *Economy and Society*, 44(2): 165–187. www.tandfonline.com/doi/abs/10.1080/03085147.2015.1013356

Vidler, A Foucault, M and Johnston, P (2014) Heterotopias. *AA Files*, (69): 18–22. www.jstor.org/stable/43202545

Wade, D and Halligan, P (2017) The biopsychosocial model of illness: a model whose time has come. *Clinical Rehabilitation*, 31(8).

Watts, S and Stenner, P (2005). Doing Q methodology: theory, method and interpretation. *Qualitative Research in Psychology*, 2: 67–91.

Watts, S and Stenner, P (2012) *Doing Q Methodological Research*. London: Sage.

Winton, A (2016) Using photography as a creative, collaborative research tool. *The Qualitative Report*, 21(2): 428–449.

PART III

Evaluating your research and understanding the wider implications

CHAPTER 12

Embedding research into practice, funding, and practicalities

Rhiannon Jones, Alice Marshall and Esme Blood

Introduction

This chapter explores *Shedding Light on Long Covid*, a research project by the Royal Society of Arts (RSA) undertaken in 2023, and the impact of effectively designed arts practice and research within public spaces by highlighting how creating new spaces for discourse allows researchers to interpret, present, and disseminate interdisciplinary research in innovative ways. S.H.E.D is a reconfigurable, D.I.Y, civic space designed to support cultural and socio-civic research practices addressing urgent societal issues. By co-designing with communities, it creates a safe space for people to discuss important issues. A Sci-Art Public Realm Research Project developed by S.H.E.D (Social Higher Education Deposit) uses the concept of a garden shed to generate dialogue in the public realm through creative placemaking. Placemaking here is defined as focusing on the local and the nuanced ways spaces are shaped by people (Courage, 2024).

Chapter concepts
- Academic research in the public realm
- Collaborating with Alumni and stakeholders
- Embodied knowledge into participatory action research
- Designing dialogue through research and practice

Ideation

S.H.E.D aims to act as a catalyst for positive change by addressing challenges such as health and wellbeing, climate crisis, economic inequalities, and promoting social mobility. In this way, it embraces a Practice as Research model (Bolt and Barnett, 2019), where practice is the key method for engagement – in this case, the engagement of clinical data by artist researchers, placed into the public realm. The main task for the artist researcher in this commissioned project by the Royal Society of Arts (RSA) was to effectively utilise scientific data and lived experience research to create an interactive

DOI: 10.4324/9781041056782-16

and immersive public experience that is co-created with patient and public representatives to highlight the challenges of Long Covid and increase public awareness. *Shedding Light on Long Covid* provided an essential platform for local and national communities to 'create together' through an ambitious creative and cultural artist-led project. In Derby, individuals had the chance to engage creatively, share lived experiences, and actively influence societal change. This was achieved by connecting people to place through artistic research and leveraging the power of the arts at policy level.

> ### Reflective question
>
> As you read this chapter, consider whether a collaborative research project with another discipline could support your own research.

Researchers and clinicians at the University of Derby approached Dr Rhiannon Jones, CEO of S.H.E.D, to ideate the project *Shedding Light on Long Covid*. They utilised S.H.E.D to bring clinical research on Long Covid into the public domain and create a national community through a creative project. Long Covid significantly impacts physical and mental wellbeing, with over 2 million people in England and Scotland affected in 2024, and around 600,000 experiencing life-altering disabilities for over three years (ONS, 2024). The project disseminated clinical research data through artistic practice and socially engaged interventions.

The project involved a design-led community initiative, with input from clinicians, patients, artists, funders, community members, and student focus groups under the curatorial stewardship of Dr. Jones. The S.H.E.D was exhibited at two sites in Derby – the Museum of Making and Derby Cathedral – to highlight health and wellbeing services in Derby through a large-scale public installation focused on Long Covid, using scientific data and lived experience research.

The research also attended to finding artistic methods to create new works that highlighted the challenges of Long Covid for patients whilst increasing public awareness. The project provided significant positive change, connecting the creative and cultural industries with the scientific community to produce a public art sculpture, unveiling new findings and impacts on society. S.H.E.D, as an artistic practice, offered insights into addressing long-term issues and living equitably with Long Covid by positioning itself as a social action model where art facilitates social engagement and change through participation (Sholette and Bass, 2018).

Top tips for new researchers:

1. If you are looking to develop a project that bridges disciplines:
    Take note of how you can use an artifact or venue to help you to facilitate a discussion and nurture a collaboration between artists and scientists. The S.H.E.D acted as an avenue to collocate people and acted as a bridge between diverse backgrounds and expertise. The outcome led to combining different perspectives in the creation of new artworks by S.H.E.D, inspired by sci-art ideas and insights being created, and put on display in the public realm space.

2. When planning your sci-art public realm project, consider how collaboration during the early ideation phase can help you uncover new research areas and formulate questions that might otherwise remain unexplored.

   Working in an interdisciplinary way can help you to challenge traditional boundaries, just as S.H.E.D did by blending artistic and scientific methods to create installations that encouraged curiosity and a deeper understanding of Long Covid.

3. Think about the civic impact of creative placemaking in your work.

   The S.H.E.D project used culture as a tool for addressing societal challenges, such as the effects of Long Covid, by building a space where clinical and academic research could be shared with the community.

4. Consider how you might design spaces or experiences that highlight important social issues, embrace public dialogue, and raise awareness.

   In this case, S.H.E.D's custom-built structure provided a platform for the lived experiences of Long Covid sufferers, offering a space for their stories to be heard while educating the public. By commissioning new works from artists that drew from both clinical and personal data, S.H.E.D not only gave visibility to Long Covid but also created a unique way for isolated patients to connect with the public, inspiring positive change.

5. As you develop your own projects, think about how you can create opportunities for dialogue and understanding.

In the Shedding Light on Long Covid project, the work facilitated positive change for isolated patients and public representatives by creating a unique platform for their voices to be heard:

> It serves as a catalyst for change, connection, and recognition. "Shedding Light on Long Covid" created the spaces needed for validation, solidarity, and empowerment by centring the narratives of those affected. Through trusting their experiences to artistic expressors, Long Covid Lived Experience Patients who collaborated in the project, could reclaim some agency over their stories ...
>
> (Sarah Barley-McMullen, Lived Experience Patient and
> Civic Champion, personal communication with
> Rhiannon Jones, 17 July 2024)

By utilising the arts to help explain the clinical research in a public setting, it lowered the barriers and increased participation and engagement with the research. Long Covid affects 7,500 people in Derby and 2.3 million nationally, posing a potential global health crisis. While most recover, 1 in 10 develop persistent symptoms, often leading to feelings of isolation and a concern of a lack of public health messaging about its long-term effects. Through the practice of research, the clinical data that was not in the public domain, and hard to interpret outside of its setting, was made accessible through artists' intervention and by the S.H.E.Ds installation design.

Clinical research had a barrier to its accessibility and lack of a public profile for whoever wanted to talk about their work in a public realm setting. However, the barrier for entry with art is lower and requires little to no prior knowledge or expertise to engage. The temporal space and place of the S.H.E.D opens access to research and clinical data to enable a wider public dialogue.

Planning

S.H.E.D is defined as a place, akin to the thinking of Michel de Certeau (1980), where a place is understood as an instantaneous configuration of multiple positions, where every element adjoins with another. Creative placemaking projects can have an interstitial function as *third spaces* (Soja, 1996) where, as grounding in an inclusive systematic approach, there is opportunity to explore and reconsider narrowly understood or ill-defined place-based situations (Courage and McKeown, 2019). This practice-led research approach fosters shared lived experiences by opening public access to research and clinical data through the temporal place and space of the S.H.E.D, placing it into the public realm for deliberation and engagement.

For the Long Covid community, funders, and the public to share their views on the design, it was continuously edited and refined, through a design-led process focused on creating new research opportunities for students, researchers, and clinicians. The role of Jones, CEO and founder of S.H.E.D, encompassed facilitating conversations, design revisions, and strategically determining the installation's placement in public settings. This included deciding where to locate the structures and commissioning creators to produce content that directly engaged with and responded to Long Covid data and patient diaries.

New researchers viewed funders as equal partners, which helped to securing funding from key stakeholders, and was critical to helping to increase visibility of the work and raise the profile. Working closely with designers Barend Slabbert and Harry Freestone, who were overseeing the build, the project curated an engaging space (Figure 12.1).

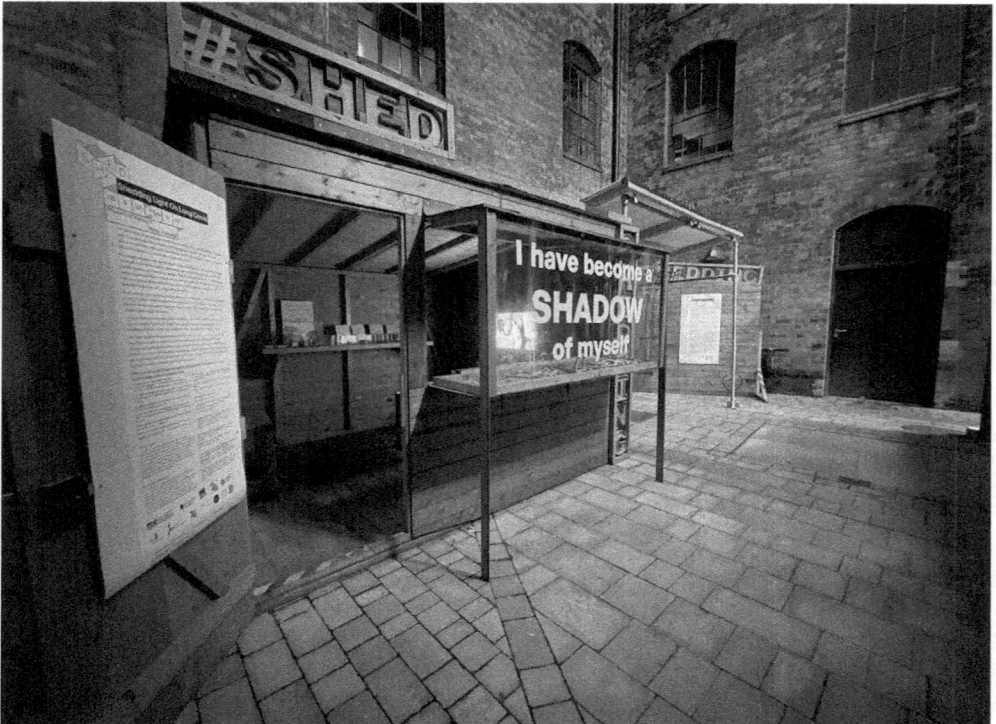

Figure 12.1 The S.H.E.D at the Museum of making

This subtle but crucial shift in language and approach significantly increased their involvement in the project, ensuring that new learnings were shared with our partners, to increase collaborative learning and engagement, and their input also fed into hearing and establishing key priorities and outcomes for the research evidenced also by the national partners: "This work provides much needed opportunities for creative practitioners to engage with new fields, experiment with their practise and engage the public with their creations" (Callum Bate, Central Area Manager for the RSA, personal communication with Rhiannon Jones, 22 July 2024).

Reflective question

Selecting the right location for your research is crucial for engaging the right communities and enriching your findings. What types of spaces would best support your research in the public realm, and why?

Integration of clinical research and artistic outputs

The range of artist researchers, including Alumni, approached to collaborate in this project was critical to ensuring an accessible and creative medium for promoting public health messages and raising awareness. Studies have shown that individuals engaged in the arts are significantly more likely to recall health messages, including sun protection, and nutrition (Mills et al, 2013). For example, public art installations, combined with social media, have been utilised to increase awareness about specific health concerns, such as the location of cardiac defibrillators (Kilaru et al, 2014). Recognising the potential of arts in health promotion, several countries, including Australia, have developed national frameworks to support the integration of arts in health and wellbeing initiatives (Davies and Pescud, 2020). These findings highlight the arts as a viable channel for communicating health messages to the general population, hence why this S.H.E.D project utilised this approach. Involving Alumni in one of the outputs helped nurture the next generation of researchers, allowing them to understand the importance of this method.

The artists involved encompassed an array of art forms, including dance, photography, spoken word, installation, and community radio. They had an open approach, ensuring that each of their processes were transparent and inviting. This resulted in an increase in participation, willingness to share lived experiences, and raised aspirations from wider community members. Combining scientific research with artistic outputs is an evolving area, yet there is a growing call for greater utilisation of this collaboration. Panhofer (2011) advocates for artistic research methodologies that incorporate embodied perceptual practices. For example, Sarkar (2020) has developed a methodology that bridges creative performance and critical research, using phenomenology and auto-ethnography to contextualise the artist's process. These approaches aim to enhance validity, build liberatory knowledge, and address epistemological concerns in conventional social psychological studies (Wasserman, 2014). With this research in mind, the use of clinical data within an artistic output will enhance methodology as well as the intended raising of the profile of Long Covid.

Using the patient diaries as a stimulus, the artist researchers produced an array of outputs. The roof of the S.H.E.D transformed into a large mouth, symbolising the vulnerability of the vessel in which Covid is tested. The Cathedral Green came alive with the voice of breathless patients, their breath carried on the wind in an immersive experience of poetry and audio. Inside the S.H.E.D, an installation prompted visitors to reflect on what Long Covid meant to them, and a live dance performance, embodying the patients' voices, guided the public audience through the Museum of Making to the S.H.E.D. Meanwhile wraparound workshop activity engaged young voices in discussions about Long Covid, creating podcasts and radio shows based on what they had learned, thereby contributing to a broader understanding of the condition.

The creative process described here is grounded in the theoretical frameworks of Embodied Knowledge and Participatory Action Research (PAR). Embodied Knowledge, rooted in phenomenology, emphasises that our bodies not only perceive but also understand in the world (Rowlands, 2013). In this project, artist researchers employed embodied practices like dance and installation art to translate the lived experiences of Long Covid patients into tangible sensory expressions. This aligns with Maurice Merleau-Ponty's (2013) theory that bodily experience is central to understanding reality, suggesting that art effectively conveys complex lived experiences.

Involving artists, researchers, and participants in this project reflects the core principles of PAR, particularly the focus on democratising knowledge production and giving a voice to those affected by Long Covid. PAR emphasises collaboration and the co-creation of knowledge (Chevalier and Buckles, 2019). By integrating patient diaries and engaging the public, this project highlights the importance of research-led practice.

This approach shows how to best leverage the relationship between clinical research and artistic practice. Engaging in this collaborative process can enhance professional development, as demonstrated by Alumni involvement, while wraparound workshops help amplify young voices and build intergenerational learning.

Reflective question

What barriers might there be for your research and how could you collaborate with artists to help with this challenge?

Case Study – Long Covid Diaries

Alice Marshall's work with Adaire to Dance has focused on character-driven storytelling to engage new audiences. Her research into character and scenario nuances has been key to making stories accessible (Marshall, 2022). **Long Covid Diaries** used this knowledge to raise public awareness of Long Covid, requiring an authentic output. Authenticity, rather than interpretation, was essential to ensure the work genuinely embodied the lived experiences it sought to convey.

The intended audience for this work was the public; in-person and online. Engaging an audience is a crucial component of raising public awareness; once engaged, the audience needs to learn and feel empowered to instigate change. Framing the work as a call-to-action laid the groundwork for future projects, with a special emphasis on Alumni involved in the project carrying this mission forward. This investigation also highlighted the importance of collaborating with partners who have an in-depth understanding of the topic, which allows for realistic clarity and transparency that is key to Embodied Knowledge being at the heart of the theoretical process (Rowlands, 2013). Having access to clinical data in the form of patient diaries allowed for this synergy.

This final performance centred around the S.H.E.D structure and the Museum of Making (Figure 12.2). The performance aimed to depict the experiences of individuals affected by the condition, emphasising the themes of solitude and communal support. The sound score incorporated excerpts from the diary entries. This integration of narrative content into the musical accompaniment sought to enhance the emotional resonance of the presentation. This approach explores narrative theory, which examines how stories and personal accounts can evoke emotional responses and create a deeper connection with the audience (Cook, 2018). The Alumni in this project actively engaged with this theory, interpreting the findings by translating the words into movement. The choreography was filmed on site providing an alternative output. The film served as a way for sheltering patients to see the work, while the live performance allowed for public engagement to boost awareness of Long Covid.

The words heard in the work are from Long Covid patients. The main method used to embody these voices is a choreographic technique called Verbatim (Paget, 2009). Verbatim is utilised across all performing arts genres, but when applied to choreography, it relies on movement to complement and enhance the spoken words. In the studio process, these words were played on a loop, focusing on three aspects:

- The rhythm
- The narrative
- The emotions

The resulting movement motif is a blend of these embodiments. The goal is not to mimic the voice but to bring the words to life. Often referred to as the universal language, dance can convey the narrative even in the absence of actual vocals, though perhaps more subjectively, the intent remains clear. This approach is crucial when engaging a public unfamiliar with a particular topic. By utilising a form of performance that can be interpreted by a diverse audience, you enhance your impact and broaden audience engagement.

The performers, all Alumni, quickly recognised their responsibility to ensure the effectiveness of this art and health sector collaboration. By integrating them into the project, it strengthened ties within the university community and showcased the transformative power of education through the Arts. Esme Blood, performer in Long Covid Diaries, now shares her insights on the project.

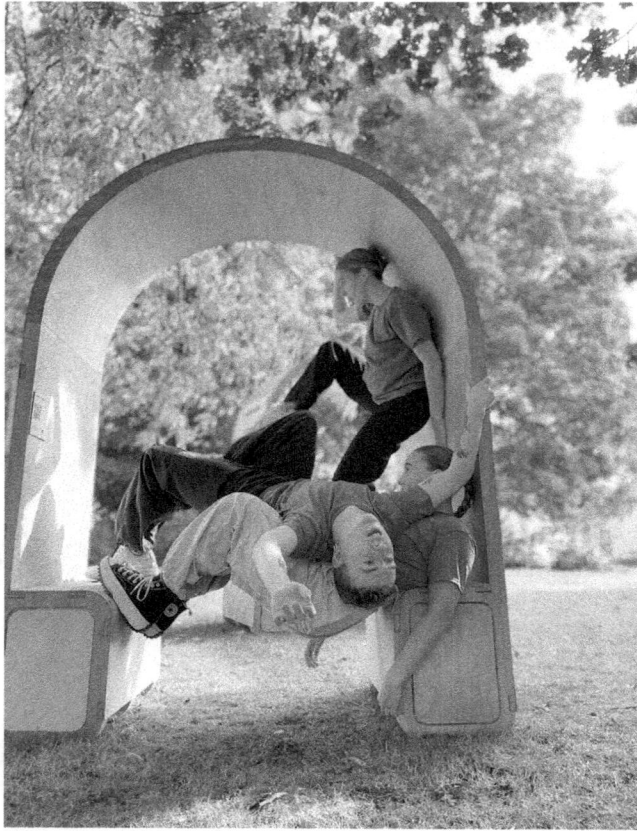

Figure 12.2 *Shedding Light on Long Covid* – Cathedral site. Dancers: Esme Blood, Charley Mitchell, Cody Jukes

Student voice

The involvement I had within the Long Covid Diaries project was both enlightening and transformative, particularly in understanding how clinical research can be embedded into artistic practice. This project was unique in that it did not merely use Long Covid as a thematic backdrop; instead, it was deeply rooted in the ongoing research surrounding the condition, making the practicalities of creation intimately tied to real-world data and lived experiences. Unlike a process that might not involve clinical research, where artistic interpretation can be more abstract or symbolic, this approach demanded a careful and respectful translation of medical findings into movement.

Through this process, I learned the importance of creating work that not only respects the factual basis of the experiences being depicted but also makes them accessible and relatable to a broader audience. The challenge was to portray the realities of Long Covid in a way that was both empathetic and accurate, without sensationalising the subject. The project's aim of raising awareness necessitated a balance between emotional engagement and factual representation, ensuring that the work was grounded in the realities faced by those with Long Covid.

Working on this project also highlighted the benefits and challenges of integrating clinical research into artistic practice. For instance, understanding the physical limitations caused by Long Covid directly influenced the movement vocabulary we developed. Alice and I had to consider how the symptoms – such as decreased energy levels – impacted the body, and this guided our creative decisions. Unlike projects that do not involve clinical research, where movement might be driven purely by aesthetic or thematic concerns, this work required a deep engagement with the medical realities of Long Covid. The movements we created needed to reflect the physical strain and energy depletion described in the symptom diaries, resulting in a unique and informed choreographic language.

The decision to capture the movement on video also stemmed from the practicalities of clinical research. Making the performance accessible to a wider audience through digital means mirrors the inclusive goals of health research, which seeks to disseminate knowledge broadly. This approach not only extended the reach of our work but also aligned with the project's aim to spread awareness about Long Covid in a manner that is both accessible and impactful.

As an Alumni, I can see how this project has significantly influenced my approach to creating movement. Prior to this, I had not engaged with a health topic as a basis for choreography, and this experience has expanded my understanding of how clinical research can inform and enhance artistic practice. The Long Covid Diaries project was an ongoing learning experience, one that will undoubtedly shape my future work, whether with Alice or other choreographers. I have seen firsthand the power of using art as a platform for education and awareness, and this has impacted how I want to present experiences through dance moving forward.

Outcomes and influences

Dialogue-based, socially engaged art forms shift away from the tradition of object-making, embracing instead a performative, process-driven approach. These practices centre on the creative orchestration of collaborative encounters and conversations, often extending well beyond the confines of institutional boundaries (Kester, 2004).

What is clear, is that *Shedding Light on Long Covid* has provided a unique space designed specifically for talking about Long Covid and that has impacted on the local cultural, social, and political discourses in Derby This project addressed the need to create a space for civic dialogue and social cohesion in relation to Long Covid. It provided both a literal and metaphorical platform for people in our city to share their experiences and perspectives. Additionally, it created opportunities for students and artist researchers to showcase their artistic talents while voicing their views on this pressing issue and others that matter to them. By embedding research into practice, the project ensured these voices were heard, generating meaningful engagement and collaboration. This is underlined by 'an irreplaceable and unique role – that Universities have – in helping their host communities to thrive – and their own success is bound up with the success of the places that gave birth to them...' (Kerslake, 2019, p 5).

How we developed community-engaged public research
You can use Table 12.1 as a skeleton for the progression of your own work.

Table 12.1 Guidance for community-engaged public research

Activity	Impact
Build a co-designed public exhibition.	Showcase scientific data and lived experience research in public realm.
Generate a public experience that is co-created with patient and public representatives.	Highlight the challenges and increase public awareness.
Attend to series of KPIs: increased health and wellbeing for Long Covid patients, improved patient experience.	Establish potential long-term collaboration with NHS through creative project.
Provide an essential platform for Long Covid lived experiences.	Actively affect societal change and engage with key stakeholders and policy makers, artists, clinicians, and academics.
Establish a partnership working group with stakeholders of the organisations.	Break the traditional working in silo but need to meet and collaborate and can do so through this project.
Engage with the public through workshops from partner.	Increase public and partner which profiles the need and engagement of project.
This interdisciplinary dialogue between artists, scientists, lived experience patients.	Lay the groundwork for evidence-based interventions and holistic and creative academic care models.

Conclusion

This project successfully addressed key performance indicators by integrating clinical data with artistic outputs to generate engagement and understanding. By merging health research with creative practices, it made complex information accessible to diverse audiences and laid the foundation for potential long-term collaboration with the NHS. This innovative, interdisciplinary approach showcased how creative methodologies can address pressing health challenges.

The initiative provided a platform for expressing the lived experiences of Long Covid patients, transforming their narratives into artistic formats that engaged stakeholders such as policymakers, clinicians, and academics. By establishing a dynamic partnership working group, the project broke traditional silos and amplified its impact, fostering connections across disciplines and sectors.

Interactive workshops conducted by project partners played a pivotal role in raising awareness and catalysing meaningful public engagement. These efforts created solidarity within the Long Covid community. As Civic Champion Sarah Barley-McMullen reflected:

> Shedding Light on Long Covid helped maintain momentum in raising awareness about Long Covid and the need for continued research, messaging, and support. By keeping the issue in the public eye and engaging policymakers, healthcare professionals, and the wider community, we advocated for increased resources and support services.
>
> (Sarah Barley-McMullen, Lived Experience
> Patient and Civic Champion, personal communication
> with Rhiannon Jones, 17 July 2024)

Integrating art with clinical research proved effective, offering an approachable way to raise awareness. This interdisciplinary approach enriched public engagement and demonstrated how blending art, science, and lived experiences can create societal impact. By prioritising collaboration, researchers can ensure their work addresses real-world challenges, inspiring greater understanding and collective action.

Reflective questions

1. Which aspects of this project could you apply to your own work?
2. Could your research be applied in a public setting?
3. How can the public be involved in your research?

References

Bolt, B and Barnett, E (2019) *Practice as Research: Approaches to Creative Arts Enquiry*. London: Bloomsbury

Chevalier, JM and Buckles, DJ (2019) *Participatory Action Research: Theory and Methods for Engaged Inquiry*. Oxford: Taylor & Francis.

Cook, PJ (2018) Understanding dance through authentic choreographic and a/r/tographic experiences. In: Chemi, T and Du, X (eds) *Arts-Based Methods and Organizational Learning*. Palgrave Studies in Business, Arts and Humanities. Cham: Palgrave Macmillan, pp 115–145. https://doi.org/10.1007/978-3-319-63808-9_6

Courage, C (2024) *Placing Placemaking: Exploring What Constitutes Best Practice in UK universities*. National Centre for Academic and Cultural Exchange. Available at: https://ncace. ac.uk/wp-content/uploads/2024/02/NCACE_Essay_ExploringPlacemaking.pdf (accessed 1 April 2025).

Courage, C and McKeown, A (2019) *Creative Placemaking. Research, Theory and Practice*. Oxford: Routledge.

Davies, CR and Pescud, M (2020) *The Arts and Creative Industries in Health Promotion: An Evidence Check Rapid Review brokered by the Sax Institute for The Victorian Health Promotion Foundation*. Ultimo, New South Wales. doi:10.57022/rdac1868.

de Certeau, M (1980) *The Practice of Everyday Life*. California: University of California Press

Kerslake, B (2019) *Truly Civic Report*. UPP Foundation.

Kester, G (2004) *Conversation Pieces: Community and Communication in Modern Art*. California: University of California Press

Kilaru, AS Asch, DA Sellers, A and Merchant, RM (2014) Promoting public health through public art in the digital age. *American Journal of Public Health*, 104: 9.

Marshall, A (2022) *Entertainment in the Performing Arts*. Oxford: Routledge.

Merleau-Ponty, M (2013) *Phenomenology of Perception*. Oxford: Taylor & Francis.

Mills, C Knuiman, MW Rosenberg, M Wood, L and Ferguson, RN (2013) Are the arts an effective setting for promoting health messages? *Perspectives in Public Health*, 133.

ONS (Office for National Statistics) (2024) *Self-Reported Coronavirus (COVID-19) Infections and Associated Symptoms, England and Scotland: November 2023 to March 2024*. Available at: www.ons.gov.uk/peoplepopulationandcommunity/healthandsocialcare/conditionsanddiseases/articles/selfreportedcoronaviruscovid19infectionsandassociatedsymptomsenglandandscotland/november2023tomarch2024 (accessed 1 April 2025).

Paget, D (2009) *New Theatre Quarterly*, 3(12): 317–336.

Panhofer, H (2011) Languaged and non-languaged ways of knowing in counselling and psychotherapy. *British Journal of Guidance and Counselling*, 39: 455–470.

Rowlands, M (2013) *The New Science of the Mind: From Extended Mind to Embodied Phenomenology*. United Kingdom: Penguin Random House LLC.

Sarkar, A (2020) Seeking theory-practice relations between humanities and fine-arts through practice of painting. *Rupkatha Journal on Interdisciplinary Studies in Humanities*, 12.

Sholette, G and Bass, C (2018) *Art as Social Action: An Introduction to the Principles and Practices of Teaching Social Practice Art*. New York: Allworth Press.

Soja, EW (1996) *Thirdspace: Journeys to Los Angeles and Other Real-and-Imagined Places*. United Kingdom: Wiley.

Wasserman, JA (2014) On art and science: an epistemic framework for integrating social science and clinical medicine. *The Journal of Medicine and Philosophy*, 39(3): 279–303.

CHAPTER 13

Analysing and disseminating the data

Tessa Godfrey, Jenni Guthrie, Rachel Watts and Charlotte Domanski

Introduction

It is not uncommon to complete your data-gathering stage and suddenly have a large and perhaps confusing amount of information in front of you that offers up more questions than answers. Data analysis, which is the process of making sense of all the information and 'data' gathered while conducting research, perhaps represents one of the greatest intellectual challenges for researchers in health and social care. However, it also offers the opportunity for creative approaches to analysis that help you bring your key findings into the light, illuminating fascinating discoveries to apply as tangible changes to your practice. Then, when your research is concluded and written up, disseminating your findings presents another important challenge and the chance for your research to help and support others in their practice journeys, and not least to help show your participants how valued and important their voices have been in your research. This chapter introduces the role of analysis and dissemination in health and social care research. We provide some practical examples of how student researchers might address these important stages of the research process, within a particular methodology (first-person action research) while exploring some theoretical frameworks that underpin analysis and dissemination.

Chapter concepts
The chapter addresses three aspects of analysis in health and social care research:

- Action research analysis in social care and health research.
- Reflexive and collaborative approaches to analysis.
- Dissemination.

DOI: 10.4324/9781041056782-17

Reflective question

As you read this chapter, we suggest that you reflect on the following:

Power is held by a researcher as they analyse and disseminate research data through the choices they make in how they represent and prioritise their participants' ideas and voices. As a researcher in the field of health and social care, how might you manage your power in an ethical and responsible manner?

Analysis in social care and health research

What is analysis?

Research involves the generation of 'data' through a variety of methods, so data can take a multitude of forms (for more details on this, see chapters 6 and 8). Data *analysis* represents the process of organising and making sense of this data (McNiff, 2017). This aspect of the research process may feel overwhelming, particularly if large amounts of data have been generated (Etherington, 2004). Reflecting on students' experience as researchers, with this book chapter co-produced by two recent social care students, analysing your research findings can be daunting due to the many different data analysis methods available. Deciding *how* to analyse your data, therefore, is an important decision when planning and carrying out your research, and helpful to consider before starting to collect your data. While your choice will have practical implications, it will also be theoretically informed. So, we will now outline some of the theoretical positions that student researchers must consider when embarking on the data analysis process.

You may wish to start by considering whether you want to 'test' an existing theory or create your own new approach by analysing your data without a specific existing theory in mind. There are two approaches to analysis to consider here: inductive and deductive (see Figures 13.1 and 13.2). Inductive analysis is seen as working from the 'bottom-up' (Creswell, 2007), creating theory and knowledge from observation and analysis of the data. Deductive analysis, on the other hand, starts with an existing theory, tested against the data.

The distinction between inductive and deductive analysis, in basic terms, reflects the difference between quantitative and qualitative research; quantitative takes a deductive approach whereas qualitative takes an inductive approach. Some qualitative researchers, however, reject this binary, arguing instead for *reflexive* analysis (Ide and Beddoe,

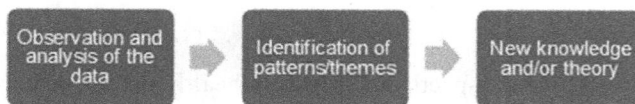

Figure 13.1 Inductive analysis

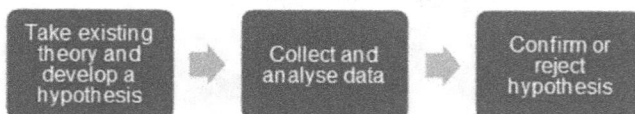

Figure 13.2 Deductive analysis

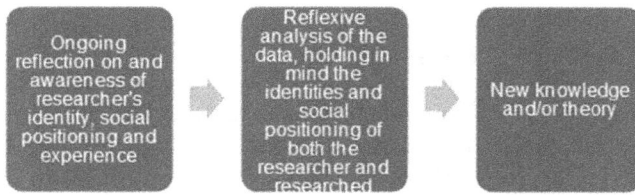

Figure 13.3 Reflective analysis

2023) in which the researcher recognises their position within the research. This approach acknowledges that researchers always bring their ideas, biases and theories to the research, influenced by a multitude of factors related to their social positioning, including race, gender, class and sexuality. These and many other characteristics will influence what they see in the data as well as the process of analysis and knowledge creation (Etherington, 2004).

How you approach analysing your data will reflect your beliefs about the nature of reality and how knowledge is acquired (Mauthner and Doucet, 2003). In research terminology, the former is referred to as the researcher's ontological position and the latter, their epistemology or epistemological position (Clark et al, 2021). Health and social care researchers conducting quantitative research, for example, might be looking for the prevalence of a particular social or health issue in a population group or wider society. For this purpose, numerical data generated in the research process will be analysed using statistical methods. This type of research represents a 'positivist' or 'realist' ontology, based on a belief that there is an objective reality separate from the researcher that can be uncovered through the process of research (Clark et al, 2021).

Qualitative research differs, with its premise being that reality is co-constructed between people and is dependent on our *interpretations* of what we observe and perceive (Creswell, 2007). There are many different approaches to analysing qualitative data, but all represent forms of interpreting data. In qualitative research it is recognised that the process of analysis is influenced by the researcher's 'conscious and unconscious' (Scheurich, 2014, p 73); their 'preconceptions, values, interests and circumstances in which they conduct the research' (Ide and Beddoe, 2023, p 727). The primary focus of this chapter is qualitative research analysis, with attention to research conducted by a group of newly qualified social workers.

Analysis in first-person action research

What is action research?

Action research is a methodology which aims to both investigate issues of social concern and address them as part of the research process. It is defined by Reason and Bradbury as:

> A participatory process concerned with developing practical knowledge in the pursuit of worthwhile human purposes... bringing together action and reflection, theory and practice in participation with others in the pursuit of practical solutions to issues of pressing concern to people.
>
> (2008, p 4)

Action research is an umbrella term which includes a variety of different types of research such as participatory, first-, second- and third-person action research. Each of these iterations reflect differences in the positioning of researcher and research participants to each other (Herr and Anderson, 2005). For example, in first-person action research, the researcher explores and makes changes in their own practice. In second-person action research, the researcher works with others to make changes to practice or organisational processes. Third-person action research seeks to influence wider social systems and therefore people who may not be known to the researcher (McNiff, 2017).

Students completing a social work master's programme have had the opportunity to undertake first-person action research, alongside working in a local authority as newly qualified social workers. They are asked to identify an area of their professional practice they want to change, so that it better aligns with their values. For example, a student might notice they avoid having discussions about race with the children and families they work with, so they may wish to improve their confidence in this area to align with their values of being an anti-oppressive and anti-discriminatory professional. With consent, students gather research data when changing their practice, during or directly after working with research participants. Data is also generated when the student gathers feedback on the changes they have made.

Analysis in first-person action research differs from analysis in more 'traditional' qualitative research. In the latter, analysis involves the researcher exploring and interpreting the meanings of the subjects of their research, being mindful of their influence on the process of analysis. This research process involves the researcher *doing something differently*, so the researcher and participant are both subjects of the research. Analysis, therefore, involves *interpreting meaning that the researcher and the participant have made together.*

In the next section of the chapter, we explore approaches students conducting first-person action research have used when analysing their data.

Reflexive and collaborative approaches to analysis

Doing first-person action research is, by nature, a self-reflexive process where students must consider the impact of the power held in the role of researcher. They must be mindful of how various aspects of their identity and experience influence the research process, and how data is analysed and thereby understood.

In addition to the focus on the self, action research is a *collaborative* methodology, where researchers do research *with people* (McNiff, 2017). This emphasis on collaboration has implications for the process of analysis, where researchers, as far as possible, should involve research participants in analysing the data. One method of analysis that enables students to involve participants in data analysis draws on the 'Coordinated Management of Meaning' (Pearce Associates, 1999).

Coordinated Management of Meaning (CMM)

CMM is 'an interpretative, critical, and practical theory of human communication underpinned by social constructionism' (Yim, 2022, p 347). Student researchers completing action research have found it to be a useful approach to adopt when analysing data because 'it offers a way to understand how people *co-construct meaning* based on their social realities and contexts' (Yim, 2022, p 347, author's emphasis).

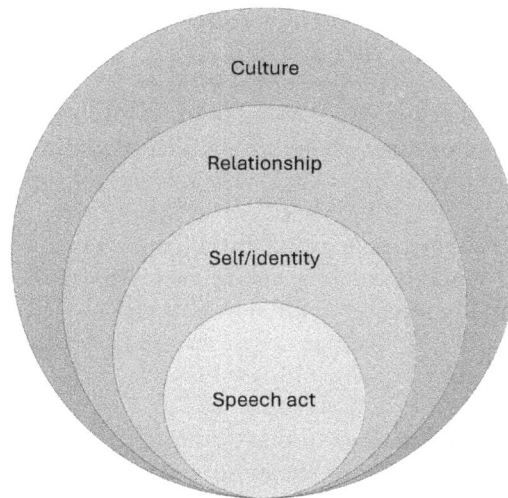

Figure 13.4 The hierarchy model

CMM provides a number of visual tools and models to facilitate the process of analysis. One of these visual tools is the hierarchy model (Figure 13.4).

To explain how this model can be used to analyse data, it is perhaps easiest to provide an example.

Simon's research

Simon is a newly qualified white British social worker. He is in his late twenties and lives with his girlfriend. He is working with Maria and her 18-month daughter Shala. Maria and Shala have mixed African-Caribbean and white heritage. Maria became a looked-after child when she was 13, when her mother became mentally unwell. Simon is working with the family due to concerns raised by the health visitor that Shala is not meeting developmental milestones, due to poor levels of care and stimulation provided by Maria.

Simon is completing first-person action research, to improve his confidence in raising concerns with parents, whilst at the same time taking a relational and anti-oppressive approach. Maria agreed to take part in the research, which she understands will involve Simon changing his practice when discussing concerns, with the opportunity for her to provide feedback on these changes.

On his last visit to Maria, Simon spoke to Maria about her strapping Shala into her buggy whilst they are in the house, which he believes may be contributing to the delay in her walking. Simon wrote up reflexive notes after the visit, forming part of his data archive. Maria agreed to analyse the following extract of data with Simon, using the hierarchy model:

When I said to Maria that children are normally walking by 18 months, Maria got upset and challenged me saying 'Are you saying she's not normal, Simon?'

The model enables Simon and Maria to consider what aspects of the hierarchy were at play during the speech act 'Are you saying she's not normal, Simon?' Maria believes that her identity as a care-experienced person informed her reaction, as this experience left her feeling 'different' and 'less than' her peers. So, Simon's suggestion that Shala is not developing in line with other children elicits feelings of 'difference' in Maria that link painfully to her past. For Simon, his identity as a newly qualified male social worker, who is not a parent, influenced his responses. While he has studied child development, his childless identity impacts on his confidence to discuss this with Maria.

They also discuss the influence of their relationship, as social worker and 'service user', particularly considering the power held in Simon's role as a social worker and researcher. As a care-experienced person, Maria has current and historical experience of the power of social workers to intervene in family life and contribute to decision making that can potentially remove children from their parents' care. Simon is mindful of the changes he is making in his practice to the relationship, aware that he must be careful to avoid harm to Maria, whilst also keeping Shala's welfare at the heart of his practice.

The model also helps Simon and Maria to consider the influence of culture on the speech act. They discuss the role of race and gender, and the potential power and oppression represented in Simon's white, male identity, which elicited feelings of anger and resistance in Maria. As a racially minoritised woman, Maria is the subject of micro- and macro-aggressions, so she experiences Simon's questioning of her parenting practices as another attack on her personhood. Together they can discuss which aspects of their context, such as their relationship and wider societal culture, were the most influential or important for them at the time.

Using the hierarchy model to analyse a small extract of data with Maria enables Simon to reflexively consider how he could mitigate for potential emotional harm to Maria, represented in his role and identity, whilst at the same time supporting Maria to care for Shala in a way that will meet all her developmental and emotional needs. Rather than coming at the end of the research process, this collaborative form of analysis can take place in the 'reflect' stage of the action research cycle, allowing Simon to make further changes to his practice based on the analysis. When writing up this analysis of the data, Simon's use of CMM allows him to incorporate Maria's analysis, as well as his own.

CMM is just one method of analysis used by students researching their practice. However, this method may not be appropriate for larger-scale research projects or research projects beyond first-person action research.

Reflexive thematic analysis

Reflexive thematic analysis (RTA) (Braun and Clarke, 2006, 2021) is a widely used method of data analysis in qualitative research. In contrast to CMM (Pearce Associates, 1999), RTA is more likely to be employed towards the end of the research process, when data generation is complete. Braun and Clarke define thematic analysis as 'a method for identifying, analysing and reporting patterns (themes) within data' (2006, p 79). A theme is identified as 'something important about the data in relation to the research question and represents some level of patterned response or meaning within the data set' (Braun and Clarke, 2006, p 82). What counts as important is influenced by the researcher, so Braun and Clarke identify their model as 'reflexive thematic analysis' (2021). They specify six stages which include 'familiarisation; generating initial codes; searching for themes; reviewing themes; refining, defining and naming themes; and writing up' (Braun and Clarke, 2006, p 87).

For students completing first-person action research, RTA has been used to make sense of the collected data as they change their practice and seek feedback. The six stages of RTA necessitate a deep and systematic engagement with data, which enables new thinking and understanding to emerge. As a method which is based on analysing data in a written form, it perhaps is less easy, though not impossible, to do collaboratively. Next, Rachel and Charlotte discuss their experience of using RTA as social work students carrying out research in their own practices.

Rachel's research

My research explored how I could better advocate for and capture the voices of non-verbal children in my practice. In order to do so, it was important to me that research focused on the voices of those I was working with, recognising their expertise through experience. This meant working with parents of the children I was supporting and colleagues I was working with within professional networks. In this way, the research data generated was collaborative – I could not conduct research without involving and drawing upon the voices of others.

When it came to analysing this data, I used thematic analysis due to its flexible approach – helpful with the subjective nature of qualitative research. I used Braun and Clarke's six-step approach to thematic analysis as described in this chapter. I used a table, looking at each of my action research cycles and 'coding' the data to look for emerging themes, identifying common occurrences across the research.

At this point, these were my ideas – my perspective of what was coming out of the research. To make this process more collaborative and remaining aligned with the action research approach, participants were involved in data analysis by offering feedback, meaning their views were directly involved in any sense of knowledge creation. This meant I would check-back about ideas and patterns I was drawing out, clarifying understanding, acting as accountability and thereby reducing the impact of a single story being told with prejudice (McNiff, 2017). These evaluations came together to shape and develop my practice with a greater sense of confidence, testing out these ideas through discussion with research participants and my student peer research group.

Charlotte's research

My research explored ways to involve extended family networks in my social work practice. Like Rachel, I also chose to use a thematic analysis approach to analyse my data as I liked the idea of using an approach that would be a good 'translator' of qualitative data that would help to draw out insights and patterns from a range of sources.

At first, I found the task of bringing all my data sources (including feedback from participants, my research notes, my reflexive journal and insights from colleagues) together a bit daunting, but I took heart from Braun and Clarke's reflection that this process can feel 'messy and organic'. I was surprised at how much data I had generated and was worried about subconsciously 'cherry picking' findings, but I found following the stages of the thematic analysis process helpful as a student researcher, as it gave me a clear steer on how to refine my findings in a methodical way.

What I particularly liked about the thematic approach was that I could place my research participants' feedback in their own words alongside my other data sources which brought their role as 'co-researchers' to life within my findings.

Dissemination

As a researcher in health and social care, it is hoped that you will have carefully designed your research in terms of approach and analysis, participant issues and ethical considerations. Similar consideration should also be given to your findings and how you intend to share your learning (Kara et al, 2021). Dissemination is generally described as a process of sharing findings relevant to your research question beyond the project itself (Kennan and Thompson, 2018; Lamont, 2021). Traditionally, academic research dissemination is through peer-reviewed journals (Chen et al, 2010). However, especially concerning participatory and practice-based research within a health and social care context, this limited scope does not equate to both research and practice ethics and values.

Ross-Hellauer et al argue that dissemination within innovative research is: 'a planned process that involves consideration of target audiences, consideration of the settings in which research findings are to be received and communicating and interacting with wider audiences in ways that will facilitate research uptake and understanding' (2020, p 1).

Thinking about action research as a methodology, we argue dissemination should be considered in line with the definition from Ross-Hellauer et al (2020) and requires a careful plan considering purpose, stakeholders, content, approach and timings.

Within health and social care research, dissemination plans need to be underpinned by a social justice approach. This is important because sharing findings with participants has not always been considered by health and social care researchers. A Canadian study of health research found that just under half (49%) did not consider dissemination (Curran et al. 2019). Purvis et al (2017) explored US research participants' experiences of receiving outcomes. They found that participants wanted to know the outcomes of research for several reasons. These included a sense of ownership of the research process, enablement of trust in researchers to engage meaningfully in the research project with them as participants and increased potential to engage in future research.

Dissemination as action

> Effective dissemination is simply about getting the findings of your research to the people who can make use of them, to maximise the benefit of the research without delay.
>
> (National Institute for Health and Care Research
> [NIHR], 2019, para 2)

Research should have a purpose and a contribution to learning for the context within which it was created. We are engaged in a process of integrating theory into practice, even if only on a small scale. In terms of first-person action research, this includes learning about your practice; however, as with all other practice-based research, others can benefit from what you have learnt. McNiff (2017) suggests action research offers a meaningful significance to the self, others we work with and the wider world. While this may seem ambitious for a student research project, understanding the potential wider impact of your research is important and relevant. It is also an invitation for creativity, to practice anti-oppressively, to advocate and to value those who made this research project happen (including you).

Who should you share your findings with?

Considering all relevant stakeholders in your research when planning your dissemination approach is important. These include your different participant groups, organisational or practice context, profession and wider stakeholders. These could include other professions and people who access health and social care services.

Thinking about your participants

The idea of trust and accountability of researchers to include participants as valued collaborators within research design is a key ethical consideration, especially if you are engaging in practice-based research (McDavitt et al, 2016). Participants have enabled your research to take place, and it is respectful and transparent to share what you have learnt with people who have offered their valuable knowledge and experience with you to achieve this. This is pertinent when the participants you involve are from groups who may be impacted by the outcomes of your research.

Rachel's experience

When it came to sharing my findings, I began by having conversations with those who took part in the research; this started within the research itself by testing out new ideas coming out of one research cycle and testing it out further by informing the next research cycle. I did this through inviting feedback from research participants, exploring their own ideas as experts through experience in this research area. Involving participants' feedback within the research helped me have a greater sense of confidence when it came to sharing my findings, knowing I had tested out ideas and made adjustments to my practice based on participants' feedback.

I subsequently shared my research in a presentation with colleagues, which helped consolidate learning and brought a sense of meaning to the project. I shared findings knowing that these ideas were formed in conversation with the families I was working with. Any sense of advocating for practice change and suggestions of better ways of working was understood through the experiences of my participants, which felt really special, particularly when thinking about the continued and often too-prevalent social exclusion of children with disabilities and their families, who were the focus of my social work practice.

My sense was that learning from and sharing findings was more meaningful due to the collaborative and reflexive journey I had gone on with my research. The research was not just about external ideas, making suggestions for simple things I could do or things I could change. There was power in the way that collaborative research meant it was not just my thoughts on this research area; there were many voices held within the views that were shared, adding a sense of accountability and value to ideas presented, elevating the experiences and expertise of the families and professionals whose voices informed and shaped all the ideas presented.

My advice to social care and health practitioners conducting research would be to remember why you chose your area of research, and to consider how you can remain aligned with this sense of purpose throughout your research. This helped me feel motivated, when sharing my findings, that this was not just about completing a project, but perhaps influencing some change in thinking and/or practice going forwards, however small.

Charlotte's experience

I also had a positive experience of sharing my findings with my research participants. I had some great moments of connection where I fed back to my participants about how their input into my research had been central to my findings and the changes I had made to my practice as a result. The participants I fed back to were really engaged with these conversations and also seemed pleased that I had listened to their ideas and feedback and could hear their own voice in my findings. It felt very rewarding to have created something meaningful in partnership with my participants and to show them how much I valued and proactively worked to understand their perspectives. Also being mindful of the main focus of my work with clients as a social worker, the feedback helped to provide a clear conclusion to my dual role as a researcher and practitioner for my participants.

I also shared my findings with my team and with another team who worked with family networks. Rather than feeling like a finite part of my research, I found that these conversations sparked more ideas for how I could continue to develop my practice even further, which helped me to realise that the cyclical nature of action research continues to live on beyond the time limits of the research project itself.

Community context

You and your participants exist within communities. Your research should benefit that community, therefore the community should be considered and included when designing your dissemination approach. The AASPIRE framework (Nicolaidis et al, 2019) (developed to enable neuro-inclusive autism research) illustrates the importance of considering both participants and researchers who are also part of the community the research is focused on. It argues that dissemination should be discussed in partnership with participants to consider what is shared, as well as when and how it is shared, to reflect the needs of that community.

Charamba and Mukurazhizha (2022) argue that in social work, failing to disseminate research into communities directly impacts practice within those communities and as such perpetuates injustice. Communities are further impacted when professionals cannot access research or develop their knowledge-based practice in an epistemologically informed way. Charamba and Mukurazhizha (2022) suggest Ubuntu principles should inform researchers' approach to dissemination. Ubuntu, a southern African philosophy, is summarily translated as 'a person is a person through others' (Mabvurira, 2020, p 74). It involves principles of relational understanding through collectivist mutual sharing, compassion, respect and humanity positions, with reciprocity both for practice and the communities it serves (Burki, 2022). Ubuntu offers an empowering approach to decolonising research beyond the white Western-centric epistemology and methodologies including participatory research (Marova and Mutanga, 2023). In essence, the research respectfully and relationally speaks with and to the communities it involves:

> The value of human relations where there is no superiority-inferiority complexity is of uttermost importance if feedback of research findings is to have a great contribution to social work practice … rather than producing rich researchers with no implementation for change to the researched individuals, groups or communities
> (Charamba and Mukurazhizha, 2022, p 182)

Putting these values into practice might involve student researchers using creative methods of dissemination that represent and respectfully connect with the relevant communities (Dierckx et al, 2023). Examples include using photography, drawings and videos to disseminate knowledge in a comprehensible and engaging way (Rose and Flynn, 2018).

Organisational context

If you are conducting research within a professional context, you will have sought ethical approval from your academic institution and/or organisational context. They may have stipulations on what and how you can share (Clark et al, 2021). This is particularly pertinent if your research is funded. You will need to ensure that you are clear regarding the parameters and permissions from organisational stakeholders in terms of what, how and when you disseminate findings.

How you plan to share findings should be explicitly included as part of your informed consent process. Consent forms should clearly list the methods of dissemination, and this should be stated within participant information forms (Clark et al, 2021). You may not share findings in all the ways you have considered, but it is harder to return to participants and ask after the project has concluded, rather than at the beginning. Curran et al (2019) note that being clear about commitment to share results responds to the research principles of beneficence and justice. Institutions should model this good practice within their information and consent templates, but responsibility also lies with researchers.

Data protection and confidentiality are key aspects to consider at this stage. For example, if you plan to include vignettes in your dissemination, you should seek consent to do this. All participants have a right to respect for their private life (Human Rights Act, 1998), which requires researchers to provide confidentiality and anonymisation (Byrne, 2016). Action research and other qualitative methods within health and social care can often involve people who access services or staff who work within these services. Some participants may be concerned they could be identified within your write-up even if you have carefully attended to pseudonyms or anonymisation of location. This may mean a potential risk to participant recruitment so student researchers should think carefully about how they can mitigate these issues, for example by excluding or changing identifying features of participants.

Turcotte-Tremblay and Mc Sween-Cadieux (2018) explored confidentiality and dissemination within West African health research and identified issues to consider when research is small scale, localised and when participants may be recognised due to their unique characteristics. They suggest participatory action research can help address the power imbalance by discussing the boundaries and risks to confidentiality, including the need to reflexively consider the impact of this on stakeholder subjectivity. This includes the impact on participants authentically sharing information within the project and what different stakeholders may want shared, especially if findings are not favourable to specific agents.

Practitioner research, such as first-person action research, requires reflexivity (Etherington, 2004) as part of data collection, analysis and consideration of findings. It can include some personal reflections and information you may not want others to read. This will require consideration of whether the dissemination of personal information or reflections might cause harm to you or others, thereby impacting on the 'beneficence' of the research – its capacity to benefit others (Herr and Anderson, 2005).

> **Reflexive questions on what to share**
>
> ■ What is the relevance for, and impact on, me and others?
> ■ How can I share my findings safely without compromising privacy?

How and when are you sharing?

Studies on research dissemination have noted that much qualitative research does not get to publication (Toews et al, 2017). Therefore, the opportunity to influence practice development is reduced. This is amplified by the current socio-political context of many health and social care organisations where resources, including time, are stretched for the busy practitioner to access and absorb research as part of their own professional development.

Dissemination plans or strategies typically consider dissemination as the '3 Ps'; publication, presentations and posters (Dudley-Brown, 2019). However, there are other ways to disseminate your findings to share learning, demonstrate your valuing of contributions and participation in your learning and contribute to the development of practice and policy. Thinking about first-person action research, the following ways to disseminate findings are suggested:

■ Through the project itself.
■ Through summaries.
■ Presentations and posters.
■ Publication.
■ Creative dissemination, through social and other media.

Through the project

The benefit of first-person action research is that there are opportunities to disseminate preliminary findings as you progress through the project. As demonstrated by Rachel and Charlotte, findings from each action cycle were shared with participants so they had a sense of how their involvement was shaping the research as well as gaining insight into their own participation. This incurs a sense of ownership and collaboration as described by Purvis et al (2017).

However, to avoid tokenistic sharing, the researcher needs to carefully ensure these findings are shared in ways that meet the needs of the participant. This includes communication preferences, accessible formats and consideration of context. For example, participants who are parents may see benefits from findings if they are linked to their own parenting situation. Colleague participants, on the other hand, may value findings that relate to their practice context. Careful use of examples to explain key themes or convey relatable messages is worth considering.

First-person action research often uses feedback from participants as data. Relating aspects of individual feedback to findings, and how you developed your practice through each cycle, can be a dissemination practice not just within your research but an approach you can assimilate into your everyday practice. Aside from dissemination through the research project itself, Table 13.1 lists additional modes of dissemination available to student researchers.

Table 13.1 Other modes of dissemination

Format	Benefits	Approach	Considerations
Summaries	An accessible way to share research findings clearly and concisely (especially for busy practitioners!).	Summaries can be shared in service newsletters, supervision or individually with participants as part of your research endings and transition back into 'practitioner mode'.	What to include in your summaries could be developed with participants so it respectfully reflects the community where your research took place. This could include translation into different languages or adapting communication styles (Charamba and Mukurazhizha, 2022; Nicolaidis et al, 2019).
Publications	The most commonly thought of method of dissemination for research, offering a broader scope of dissemination with the possibility of your research being read by a large number of people.	Time is your greatest resource if you are seeking to formally publish your research findings, which is not often available for student researchers. You may want to seek advice from your organisation on how they could support you to achieve this. Most journals have information and advice for authors which can be found on journal websites. Each journal will have its preferred approach to structure and referencing as well as timescales for publication. All peer-reviewed journals will have a process that includes reviewing your writing by at least one other academic or researcher who may remain anonymous through the process. Their feedback will offer recommendations for any amendments and can be useful for your own academic writing development.	Publishing can be a meticulous process involving editing and reviewing of your writing that may or may not eventually get accepted for publication. Considering who your audience is, and approaching journals relevant to your research focus, audience and practice context will enable your findings to be shared more effectively. Seek a mentor from your context who may have published previously to guide you through the process. Publication may not necessarily need to occur once your project is completed. There may be opportunities to disseminate aspects of your research at varying points of your project.

(Continued)

Table 13.1 (Continued)

Format	Benefits	Approach	Considerations
Creative methods	Enable your research to speak to and of the community the research represents (Keen and Todres, 2007).	Voices within research can be empowered by using methods that represent cultural aspects such as music, art or imagery.	Gameiro et al (2018) used drawing activities with women from minoritised race and religious backgrounds in the UK to discuss sensitive health issues. By using the artwork to disseminate these findings, voices remained representative of their diverse communities.
Social media	Opportunity to make research accessible to busy practitioners who need to keep up with research but may struggle to do so in pressured work contexts such as frontline health and social work teams.	A systematic review by Roberts-Lewis et al (2024) found that high frequency, multiple platforms, accessible format (imagery and blogs) and involvement of influencers offered greater potential impact.	Check your organisational social media policy and take care that the sites you use reflect your own research values.

Conclusion

Data analysis and dissemination will form separate but essential components of students' research projects. In this chapter, we have outlined some of the different forms that analysis can take and have given advice, underpinned by research evidence, on the key decisions that need to be taken when planning research dissemination. Student experiences outlined in the chapter have identified how taking a collaborative approach to both analysis and dissemination has aligned with the social justice values of social care and health research and research beneficence (Wood, 2017).

Useful resources

For student researchers in health and social care who are considering using thematic analysis for the first time, Braun and Clarke's 'Thematic Analysis: A Practical Guide' (2021) provides a helpful resource.

For students considering CMM as a method of analysis, W. Barnett Pearce's 'Making Social Worlds: A Communication Perspective' (2007) is a useful starting point. There are also a number of freely available online videos outlining CMM theory and providing an overview of the hierarchy model, used in the previous example, and other CMM models, such as the Daisy and LUUUUTT models.

The National Institute for Health and Care Research has a useful accessible guide for planning a dissemination strategy including principles of good dissemination (NIHR, 2019).

References

Braun, V and Clarke, V (2006) Using thematic analysis in psychology. *Qualitative Research in Psychology*, 3(2): 77–101.

Braun, V and Clarke, V (2021) *Thematic Analysis: A Practical Guide*. 1st Edn. Thousand Oaks: SAGE Publications.

Burki, T, (2022) Research focus: the Ubuntu Center. *The Lancet*, 400(10368): 2034.

Byrne, D (2016) *Research Ethics*. Los Angeles, CA: SAGE Publications.

Charamba, S and Mukurazhizha, R (2022) The hurdle of disseminating social work research findings in Zimbabwe and a proposed model. *African Journal of Social Work*, 12(4): 179–188.

Chen, PG Diaz, N Lucas, G and Rosenthal, MS (2010) Dissemination of results in community-based participatory research. *American Journal of Preventive Medicine*, 39(4): 372–378.

Clark, T Foster, L Bryman, A and Sloan, L (2021) *Bryman's Social Research Methods*. Oxford: Oxford University Press.

Creswell, JW (2007) *Qualitative Inquiry and Research Design: Choosing Among Five Traditions*. London: SAGE Publications.

Curran, D Kekewich, M and Foreman, T (2019) Examining the use of consent forms to promote dissemination of research results to participants. *Research Ethics*, 15(1): 1–28.

Dierckx, C Zaman, B and Hannes, K (2023) Sparking the academic curriculum with creativity: students' discourse on what matters in research dissemination practice. *Arts and Humanities in Higher Education*, 22(1): 3–25.

Dudley-Brown, S (2019) Dissemination of evidence in nursing and healthcare. In: White, KM Dudley-Brown, S and Terhaar, MF (eds) *Translation of Evidence Into Nursing and Healthcare*. New York: Springer, pp 255–267.

Etherington, K (2004) *Becoming a Reflexive Researcher: Using Ourselves in the Research*. London: Jessica Kingsley Publishers.

Gameiro, S de Guevara, BB, El Refaie, E and Payson, A (2018) Drawing out–an innovative drawing workshop method to support the generation and dissemination of research findings. *PloS one*, 13(9): e0203197.

Herr, K and Anderson, G (2005) *The Action Research Dissertation*. Los Angeles, CA: SAGE Publications.

Human Rights Act (1998), c42.

Ide, Y and Beddoe, L (2023) Challenging perspectives: reflexivity as a critical approach to qualitative social work research, *Qualitative Social Work*, 23(4): 725–740.

Kara, H Lemon, N Mannay, D and McPherson, M (2021) Dissemination. In: Kara, H et al (eds) *Creative Research Methods in Education*. Bristol: Policy Press, pp 143–158.

Keen, S and Todres, L (2007) Strategies for disseminating qualitative research findings: three exemplars. *Forum Qualitative Sozialforschung/Forum: Qualitative Social Research*, 8(3).

Kennan, MA and Thompson, K (2018) Research writing and dissemination. In: Williamson, K and Johanson, G (eds) *Research Methods: Information, Systems and Context*. Cambridge: Chandos Publishing, pp 517–532.

Lamont, T (2021) *Making Research Matter Steps to Impact for Health and Care Researchers*. Bristol: Policy Press.

Mabvurira, V (2020) Hunhu/Ubuntu philosophy as a guide for ethical decision making in social work. *African Journal of Social Work*, 10(1): 73–77.

Marovah, T and Mutanga, O (2023) Decolonising participatory research: can Ubuntu philosophy contribute something? *International Journal of Social Research Methodology*, 27(5): 501–516.

Mauthner, NS and Doucet, A (2003) Reflexive accounts and accounts of reflexivity in qualitative data analysis. *Sociology*, 37(3): 413–431.

McDavitt, B Bogart, LM Mutchler, MG Wagner, GJ Green Jr, HD Lawrence, SJ Mutepfa, K and Nogg, KA (2016) Peer reviewed: dissemination as dialogue: building trust and sharing research findings through community engagement. *Preventing Chronic Disease*, 13: E38. https://doi.org/10.5888/pcd13.150473

McNiff, J (2017) *Action Research: All You Need to Know.* London: SAGE Publications.

National Institute for Health and Care Research (NIHR) (2019) *How to Disseminate Your Research.* Available at: www.nihr.ac.uk/documents/how-to-disseminate-your-research/19951 (accessed 30 June 2024).

Nicolaidis, C, Raymaker, D Kapp, SK Baggs, A Ashkenazy, E McDonald, K Weiner, M Maslak, J Hunter, M and Joyce, A (2019) The AASPIRE practice-based guidelines for the inclusion of autistic adults in research as co-researchers and study participants. *Autism: The International Journal of Research and Practice,* 23(8): 2007–2019.

Pearce Associates (1999) *Using CMM: The Coordinated Management of Meaning.* Available at: www.scribd.com/document/396811859/doc (accessed 10 April 2025).

Pearce, WB (2007) *Making Social Worlds: A Communication Perspective.* Blackwell: London.

Purvis, RS Abraham, TH Long, CR Stewart, MK, Warmack, TS and McElfish, PA (2017) Qualitative study of participants' perceptions and preferences regarding research dissemination. *AJOB Empirical Bioethics,* 8(2): 69–74.

Reason, P and Bradbury, H (2008) *The Sage Handbook of Action Research: Participative Enquiry and Practice.* 2nd Edn. London: SAGE Publications.

Roberts-Lewis, S Baxter, H Mein, G Quirke-McFarlane, S Leggat, FJ Garner, H Powell, M White, S and Bearne, L (2024) Examining the effectiveness of social media for the dissemination of research evidence for health and social care practitioners: systematic review and meta-analysis. *Journal of Medical Internet Research,* 26: e51418.

Rose, C and Flynn, C (2018) Animating social work research findings: a case study of research dissemination to benefit marginalized young people. *Visual Communications,* 17(1): 25–46.

Ross-Hellauer, T Tennant, JP Banelytė, V, Gorogh, E Luzi, D Kraker, P Pisacane, L Ruggieri, R Sifacaki, E and Vignoli, M (2020) Ten simple rules for innovative dissemination of research. *PLoS Computational Biology,* 16(4): p.e1007704.

Scheurich, JJ (2014) *Research Method in the Postmodern.* London: Routledge.

Toews, I Booth, A Berg, RC Lewin, S Glenton, C Munthe-Kaas, HM Noyes, J Schroter, S and Meerpohl, JJ (2017) Dissemination bias in qualitative research: conceptual considerations. *Journal of Clinical Epidemiology,* 88: 133–139.

Turcotte-Tremblay, AM and Mc Sween-Cadieux, E (2018) A reflection on the challenge of protecting confidentiality of participants while disseminating research results locally. *BMC Medical Ethics,* 19: 5–11.

Wood, L (2017) The ethical implications of community-based research: a call to rethink current review board requirements. *International Journal of Qualitative Methods,* 16: 1–7.

Yim, S (2022) A critique of coordinated management of meaning and circularity in relation to countering oppressive practice: reflections from a trainee therapist. *Australian and New Zealand Journal of Family Therapy,* 43(3).

CHAPTER 14

The holistic nature of health and social care

Antonette Hall and Robin Sturman-Coombs

Introduction

This chapter explores the holistic nature of health and social care. Holistic means exploring the physical, psychological, and sociological aspects of individuals and how these are influenced by the delivery of health and social care services. We consider how these systems interact, often causing conflict, complexities, and controversy (Crotty, 1998). This chapter explores the influence of the political climate and the unique experiences of individuals from global ethnic majority backgrounds. We also provide a definition and contextual understanding of the holistic nature of health and social care, highlighting its connections to related areas such as education, housing, and poverty.

Chapter concepts
■ Defining the holistic nature of health and social care
■ Impact of social determinates on health and well-being
■ Political, economic, and social climate of health and social care

Defining 'holistic nature of health and social care'
The World Health Organization (WHO) defines health as holistic and positive, considering it is a 'state of complete physical, mental and social well-being and not merely the absence of disease or infirmity' (WHO, 2025). This definition links health with well-being, framing it as a fundamental human right that necessitates physical and social resources for attainment and maintenance (Faculty of Public Health, 2024). The WHO's definition has been criticised as inadequate when addressing contemporary challenges. Leonardi (2018) and Huber et al (2016) argued that the term 'complete state of well-being' is problematic as it implies absoluteness, which is difficult to measure as individuals will encounter physical and mental challenges in their lifetime. This definition does not account for individuals with disabilities who may perceive themselves as healthy (Schramme, 2023), overlooking the temporary state of ill health and people living with chronic illnesses (Martino, 2022).

DOI: 10.4324/9781041056782-18

McCartney et al (2019) assert health is a 'state of being', allowing them to experience pain or enjoy positive mental well-being. For an individual or group to achieve complete physical, mental, and social well-being, they must be able to identify and cope with their surroundings. Thus, health can be seen as the resource necessary to function in everyday life and not the goal of living (WHO, 2025). As such, systems, environments, and policies should support an individual's health (Shilton et al, 2011). Health is a positive concept of social and personal resources and physical capacities allowing individuals to function in society. Positive and negative health exists not as a dichotomy, but as a continuum. Therefore, the absence of disease or disability is neither sufficient nor necessary for good health (Card, 2017). Health is socially determined by factors located in different levels of society, ranging from the individual to the structural systems (Dahlgren and Whitehead, 2006), which impact people's life outcomes.

The term social care has no legal definition (Mind UK, 2018); however, it can be described as the service providing a safety net to those at risk and empowers them to participate in society (The King's Fund, 2024). Social care has been overseen by local authorities with different democratically elected governance structures. While they adhere to national policy, local authorities have more autonomy in determining how to implement policies and allocate funding. Collaborative efforts between health and social care are necessary, yet despite efforts to integrate health and social care, there is a twofold divide (Iliffe and Manthorpe, 2014), thus promoting inequity (The King's Fund, 2024).

The ambiguity surrounding the definitions of health and social care can pose challenges for students when it comes to defining the scope of their research; students should clearly define their key terms and delineate the boundaries of their research topic.

The political climate of health and social care

The political climate impacts health and social care services, affecting their delivery and how they are experienced by service users (Wang et al, 2018). This section will consider three principal themes regarding the political climate of health and social care. It first considers the ongoing effect of the *Covid years*, followed by the impact and role of the 'Welfare State' and then finally consideration of health and social care for the Global Ethnic Majority (GEM) and Widening Participation (WP).

For many years researchers, practitioners, academics, and politicians have argued in favour of wedding health and social care systems more neatly together to meet the holistic needs and nature of individuals (Mercer et al, 2021). Why this has not happened remains a widely contested debate, with a plethora of reasons being offered. However, the Covid pandemic of 2019, and what followed, evidences clearly the need for joint working (Department of Health and Social Care [DHSC], 2022). The pandemic itself was responsible for a range of direct and indirect impacts on public health, mental well-being, economic stability, social interactions, and access to essential services. It affected healthcare systems, increased social and health inequalities, disrupted education, and altered daily life for people worldwide (DHSC, 2022). Covid left a legacy of patients missing appointments and referrals (DHSC, 2022). The indirect effects have been equally harmful and impactful. The Covid pandemic compounded the already high pressures in the social care system and many social care services felt abandoned (King's College London, 2020). Covid resulted in many individuals being profoundly affected, with delays in speech and language development for newborns (Royal College of Speech and Language Therapists, 2022) to early preventable deaths for older citizens (Pearson-Stuttard et al, 2023). For many, the outlook remains bleak, underscoring the essential role of the welfare state.

The welfare state

The delivery of the welfare state, according to Garland (2021), should be a principle of any democracy in which a safety net should be provided should individuals *fall on hard times*. Its purpose is to meet the fundamental and holistic needs of individuals and plays a crucial role in promoting the holistic nature of health and social care by ensuring that comprehensive support systems are in place for all (Pailer et al, 2022). It integrates various services, such as healthcare, social services, and financial support, to address the diverse needs of the population. By providing a safety net through public health programmes, social security, and welfare benefits, the welfare state ensures that individuals receive not only healthcare but also support for social determinants of health, such as housing, education, and employment (Moller and Cai, 2020). This comprehensive approach advances overall well-being and underscores the interconnectedness of physical, mental, and social health. Though the focus is on the provision of holistic care, sadly the welfare state has created, rather than addressed, divisions within society (Titmuss, 2018).

This division in how individuals are viewed is not a recent phenomenon; welfare is sadly wrapped up in the language of division (Garland, 2021). This creates a harmful narrative that separates and stigmatises individuals based on their need for assistance, rather than fostering a unified and supportive society (Garland, 2021). The welfare state is under intense political scrutiny due to a range of factors, including economic pressures that raise concerns about the affordability and sustainability of welfare programmes (Taylor-Gooby et al, 2017). The Coalition Government, in 2010, officially announced a period of austerity and a desire to roll back the welfare state (Bochel and Powell, 2016). For some, the welfare state has become an oppressive tool that acts not to support and help the individuals but to punish and scorn them for needing the support of the welfare state (Gibbs and Lehtonen, 2019). The evocative film 'I Daniel Blake' represents this paradox (Loach, 2016). It depicts the inhumane and panoptic view that central Government has adopted in the delivery of the welfare state. This is not, however, simply a dramatised film. The welfare state has seen exceptional funding cuts since 2010, with record levels of money being diverted away from Local Government Services. In 2023 it was reported that 'The average council now faces a £33m predicted deficit by 2025–26- a rise of 60% from £20m two years ago' (Tomas and Lynch, 2023).

Several Local Authorities have unprecedently declared themselves bankrupt (Tomas and Lynch, 2023). Therefore, meeting fundamental individual needs has become profoundly challenging for families, echoed in the rise in food banks and children being referred to children services (Sosenko et al, 2022). If the role of the welfare state was to ensure that individuals can *fare well*, we must question its true purpose. Thus, the impact is not what was initially intended. The welfare state is pivotal in delivering health and social care services by integrating comprehensive and complex systems that address the diverse and interconnected needs of individuals, thereby promoting holistic well-being. This section underscores the significance of students understanding the political, social, and economic climate when undertaking research. This is because research must be adaptive and responsive to the presenting needs of a society. The following section considers this in the wider context of an individual's education and housing needs alongside the role of poverty.

Education, poverty, housing, and health and social care

It is essential to comprehend the relationship between education and health, as it is crucial for reducing health disparities and enhancing individual well-being (Zajacova and Lawrence, 2018). How education affects health is complex and interlaced, as the distribution and content of education changes over time (Lynch, 2003). Research suggests that the link between low educational attainment and poor health can be attributed to various socioeconomic factors (Raghupathi and Raghupathi, 2020). As a result, it is argued that better education leads to better, more stable jobs that pay higher incomes and allow families to accumulate wealth that can be used to improve health. Economic factors are equally an important link to education and health outcomes, accounting for 30% of the correlation (Mirowsky, 2017). Consequently, education is recognised as a crucial social determinant of health (Ro et al, 2016). According to WHO (2024) a social determinant of health are non-medical factors that impact health outcomes. They include circumstances in which individuals are born, grow, work, and live. These are influenced by wider systems such as economic policies, development agendas, and social policies that shape daily life. However, despite these assertions, macro-level politics influence and shape social and health disparities that affect educational attainment.

These widening gaps in society are avoidable, and alterations in the relationship between education and health are closely tied to social policies (Zajacova and Lawerence, 2018). Furthermore, the Marmot Review (2010) draws parallels between educational and health inequalities, emphasising that both are persistent factors contributing to broader social disparities for ethnic groups (Parliament UK, 2010, p 25).

Multiple studies have investigated the socioeconomic disparity in health across the UK and several Nordic countries, having concluded that education and occupational class are contributing factors to health inequalities (Huijts et al, 2010). Zimmerman and Woolf (2024) argued that education plays a pivotal role in shaping health outcomes and promoting well-being in society. They further concluded that education is a driving force at each ecological level. Consequently, individuals with access to quality education are equipped with knowledge and skills to make informed choices about their health when compared to their less educated counterparts. Moreover, education fosters critical thinking and problem-solving abilities, which are essential for navigating health and social care systems. By empowering individuals to adopt healthy behaviours and lifestyles, education ultimately contributes to better health overall and increased life expectancy (Mirowsky, 2017).

These educational disparities and unequal life expectancy rates are concerning and necessitate attention. Furthermore, the presence of housing discrepancies linked to race/ethnic background and other social factors raises moral dilemmas and contradicts the core principles of equity and justice in society (Whitehead, 1992; Sen et al, 2004). Thus, although it is a basic human right (Equality and Human Rights Commission [EHRC], 2023) for individuals to live in warm, secure, and decent homes, and to be treated with dignity and equality, many people in England live in houses that are considered less decent which may put their health at risk or even death (GOV UK, 2024). In England, the relationship between poor housing tenure and health can be explained by the inferior internal housing conditions and increased problems associated with social housing (Macintyre et al, 2003). In 2020, two-year-old Awaab Ishak died from serious respiratory infection caused by continued exposure to damp and mould from living in poor social housing conditions. The coroner reported that this was a case of a catalogue of failures (GOV UK, 2024). The BRE trust published The Cost of Poor Housing research, which defines poor housing as a 'dwelling that fails to meet the statutory minimum standard of housing needs in England' (Garrett et al, 2021, p 7). Furthermore, the independent Marmot Review (2010) described housing as a social determinant of health, recognising how a lack of housing or poor-quality housing can negatively affect health and well-being, increasing inequalities throughout life.

In the UK, it is estimated that one in five people live in poverty, adversely impacting an individual's holistic well-being (Liaqat et al, 2021) and increasing health disparities and barriers in accessing health and social care services (The King's Fund, 2024). However, as the concept of poverty is contested, ways of measuring poverty are also disputed and therefore varied. The King's Fund (2024) indicated that a social gradient demonstrates that a person's socio-economic position is linked to their health. This association begins in childhood, with the poorest experiencing the highest rates of infant mortality. This trend continues into adulthood, as people who experience poverty throughout their lives are more likely to die at a younger age (World Population Review, 2021). This creates a gap of more than 20 years in life expectancy between people living in most and least deprived areas (Dwyer-Lindgren et al, 2017). It is important to note that the number of children living in poverty in the UK has risen, which the United Nations characterised as 'not just a disgrace, but a social calamity and an economic disaster, all rolled into one' (Alston, 2018). Concurrently, the resources available to health and social care services have diminished, constraining their ability to address these negative trends such as the rise in poverty (Cooper and Stewart, 2013). The need to integrate the consequences of these negative trends into a student's research journey cannot be stated enough.

Policy and legislation context framework

In the UK, studies (Raleigh, 2023; Dunn et al, 2022) have indicated that health and social care services are under extreme pressure with a growing number of individuals struggling to access the care they need to participate fully in society. Nonetheless, policymakers, researchers, and public health practitioners have been steadfast in their efforts to not only enhance overall population health but also to minimise or eradicate health disparities stemming from geography, race/ethnicity, socioeconomic status, and other social factors (Braveman et al, 2011). As a result, the Health and Care Act (2022) brought significant changes to the regulations and framework of the National Health Service (NHS) in England, reversing elements of the market-focused reforms implemented by the Coalition Government ten years earlier. According to Dunn et al (2022), these changes are founded on the belief that collaboration across different sectors is essential for enhancing health outcomes and addressing health disparities. Similarly, the integrated care systems were implemented by national policymakers to reduce health inequalities enhancing a joined-up approach with health and social care services, ensuring that people get the support they need, at the right place and time.

More recently, the pandemic has exacerbated these health inequalities and pressures on health and social care services (Dunn et al, 2022). These issues built upon a longstanding history of policies promoting cross-sector collaboration in healthcare and social care (Anderson et al, 2022; Alley et al, 2016). Nonetheless, translating national policy into local action is challenging as health inequalities are complex issues; thus, policy objectives to reduce them are often ambiguous, unclear, and incomplete (Ford et al, 2021). Similarly, many researchers suggest that a lack of clarity on policy aims and objectives delays collaboration between local agencies, which are expected to work together to deliver them (Alderwick et al, 2022). To create impactful public policies, it is essential to establish clear and contextually relevant operational definitions. These definitions enable the setting of objectives and specific targets, prioritisation of limited resources, and evaluation of progress. Clear definitions are particularly crucial given the lack of advancement in reducing disparities in health and social care based on race/ethnicity and socioeconomic status (Braveman and Egerter, 2008).

Furthermore, ethnic minority groups, older people, and those from socially deprived areas have experienced many challenges and inequalities in accessing health and social care services (The King's Fund, 2024). Health inequalities in the UK have continued to widen, further exacerbating existing disparities. These have resulted in widespread criticism of the country's policies and policymakers, indicating a multi-level failure to protect the most vulnerable members of society, addressing longstanding and historical issues (Bambra, 2012; Barr et al, 2012; Thomas et al, 2010; Thorlby and Maybin, 2010). The DHSC (2024) emphasises the need for all parts of the NHS, public health, and social care system to actively connect, communicate, and collaborate. Moreover, the Social Care Institute of Excellence (2014) placed importance on an individual's overall welfare, requiring decision-making and planning to prioritise their well-being over specific service-related needs (UK Government, 2022). The Health and Care Act (2022) has introduced a new legislative measure to foster collaboration between the health and social care sectors to address inequalities and cater to the diverse needs of individuals requiring multiple services (The King's Fund, 2022). As a result, the government has launched the 'Levelling Up Health' mission to enhance healthy life expectancy and reduce health inequality gaps. This initiative has been praised for recognising the importance of addressing health disparities and improving overall quality of life, potentially extending an individual's lifespan by up to five years (Dunn et al, 2022). Despite these positive developments, some researchers have noted that the current agenda lacks distinctiveness compared to previous efforts to reduce regional inequalities (Tomaney and Pike, 2020). The health disparities white paper has faced criticism for impeding progress in addressing health inequalities and for not adequately addressing the factors influencing health and contributing to inequality. For instance, it fails to consider early life experiences, educational outcomes, housing needs, and income disparities (Dunn et al, 2022).

Policies play a crucial role in shaping research, particularly in academic contexts, as they provide a framework that guides the research process and its outcomes. Therefore, policies are a fundamental factor that shape the direction, scope, and ethics of any research. For students, comprehending and navigating the diverse array of policies are essential for successfully conducting research that is not only rigorous and ethical, but also aligned with wider institutional and societal objectives. Although policies can offer valuable guidance and support, they can also impose constraints that challenge students to be innovative and resourceful in the research journey.

Widening Participation and Global Ethnic Majority outcomes
in the context of health and social care

In the context of discussing the holistic nature of health and social care, promoting Widening Participation (WP) and enhancing outcomes for Global Ethnic Majority (GEM) communities are imperative if we are to create a society that values equity and fairness (Equality and Human Rights Commission, 2023). Whilst, according to the Universal Declaration of Human Rights (United Nations General Assembly, 1948) 'we are all born free', we know that individuals from a range of GEM and many WP backgrounds do not experience the same trajectories, outcomes, and longevity that white communities do. Several national and global events have brought into sharp focus the discriminatory and unequal treatment faced by many GEM communities. The death of George Floyd in the US amplified already and understandably frustrated communities who repeatedly observed the inhuman treatment of non-white communities (Macleod, 2018). The Grenfell Tower disaster in the UK further amplified and ignited communities tired with the inequalities and social disparities (Lussenhop, 2020).

Women in the poorest 10% of areas in England can expect to live on average 78.7 years. In contrast, women living in the richest 10% of areas in England have an average life expectancy of 86.4 years (Child Poverty Action Group, 2022). Children from the poorest backgrounds are 17 times more likely to end up in care compared to those from the wealthiest backgrounds (Bywaters et al, 2023). These stark disparities highlight the profound impact of socioeconomic status on the lives and futures of children. It underscores the urgent need for family centred interventions and supportive measures to address the root causes of poverty and provide equitable opportunities for all children, regardless of their socioeconomic background. Disparities in outcome are not, however, just observed between geographical locations. There are distinct differences and disparities between ethnic and racial groups (Kapadia et al, 2022). Raleigh (2023) reported that some of the worst health outcomes are observed in White Gypsy or Irish Traveller, Bangladeshi and Pakistani communities, by comparison to white communities. With a focus on the Early Years, infant and maternal mortality are profoundly higher among Black and South Asian groups than white groups (Raleigh, 2023). In comparison there are distinct health issues amongst white communities, notably Alzheimer's, cancer, and dementia. However, these outcomes need not be the case if a greater focus was placed on the early years of life.

The first 1001 critical days present an opportunity to have the greatest effect on an individual's short-, medium-, and long-term outcome. Kapadia et al (2022) demonstrate the importance of investing in the Early Years and maternity care. Their research evidenced that women from ethnic minorities were at greater risk during childbirth, with Black women four times more likely to die than other racial or ethnic groups. Asian women were twice as likely and those women living in deprived areas were three times more likely to die in childbirth than non-deprived communities. The Institute for Fiscal Studies (2022) also identified a relationship between race and infant mortality linking health and social care outcomes to the economic success of communities, with poorer and more disadvantaged communities experiencing greater degrees of health inequalities (Mirza and Warwick, 2022). Focusing on enhancing the rights of Global Ethnic Majority (GEM) communities within the broader agenda of health and social care is essential for promoting equity and inclusivity (EHRC, 2023). By prioritising their rights systemically, society can address these inequalities, ensure fair access to quality care, and improve health outcomes. This approach fosters a more just society and enriches the healthcare system by incorporating diverse perspectives and needs. The emphasis on creating enriching and fair health and social care systems must start at the point an individual embarks on their research and student journey, not simply when services are delivered.

Student voice

During my master's research project, I delved into the investigation of Black Female Staff and Student Identity: Progression, Race, and Equality within Higher Education in Britain. The study aimed to explore the influence of identity, race, and equality on the career progression of Black females. It involved a critical examination and analysis of the perspectives and lived experiences of Black female students and staff from various universities and courses, focusing on their career progression, identity, race, equality, and university systems and structures. Whether research is undertaken by an academic or a student, it is fundamental for creating change within various contexts. Despite the availability of well-documented research throughout history, continued research is essential for addressing existing issues and understanding what, why, and how of phenomena and their impact. Identifying a gap in the research field can set one's research apart. As a student, choosing a topic and research area that one is passionate about is crucial, as it can drive impactful change. A comprehensive study involves conducting both primary and secondary research, which are fundamental to the research process.

The process can be challenging and time-consuming, so managing your time is crucial. Start by brainstorming and creating a list of keywords, as this will help to focus your research on your chosen topic. I utilised a variety of sources, including books, journals, questionnaires, and semi-structured interviews, to conduct my research. In reflecting on my recent research, I particularly enjoyed primary research because there is something powerful about hearing people's voices and capturing their lived experiences. Conducting primary research allows for the collection of rich and authentic data, which can shine a light on areas of racial, social, educational, and health inequalities and the persistent systemic barriers that disempower under-represented groups. I am driven to pursue research because I believe it has the potential to break down barriers, influence policies and practices, and ultimately eradicate inequalities across all institutions. The most valuable lesson I have learned at the University is that key research findings can inform and shape policies, drive social change, establish effective practices, and promote equal opportunities and equity in institutions and wider contexts. As a student researcher, choosing your research method is crucial, it provides insights into the chosen subject area, fostering a deeper understanding of the research process, developing research questions, and testing hypotheses from an unbiased perspective. It's important to pilot test and address your research questions, as this stage is critical in identifying any potential issues before the full study commences. Transcribing the data can be time-consuming so use thematic analysis to identify common themes, trends, and patterns within your qualitative data. This approach has assisted me in identifying codes and capturing compelling aspects of the data that are appropriate to the research question.

Conclusion and next steps

This chapter has considered and explored the holistic nature of health and social care. It has critiqued the impact and role of policy and law on the day to day lived experiences of individuals and communities. This chapter presents several findings. Firstly, health and social care inequalities are predominantly observed in deprived and Global Ethnic Majority (GEM) communities. Secondly, the Covid-19 pandemic, poor housing, and education and poverty have exacerbated these disparities, profoundly impacting these groups. Thirdly, fiscal decisions and the political climate have further affected the delivery of the welfare state, often limiting access to essential services. Thus, ensuring the right decisions are made in the Early Years is crucial, as these can have a profound medium- to long-term impact on the well-being of infants, children, adults, families, and communities, fostering more equitable and supportive environments. Despite the moderately bleak picture presented in this chapter, there must always be hope and aspiration for a better future. We view students as key to addressing these inequalities, through policy, practice, and research.

Reflective questions

1. How does access to quality education influence long-term health outcomes?
2. In what ways do housing affordability and stability influence health inequalities?
3. How might the intersection of poverty with other factors like race, gender, or disability lead to compounded health inequalities?
4. How does your own experience or observation of education, housing, and poverty shape your understanding of health inequalities?
5. In what ways do policies addressing social determinants of health (education, housing, poverty, employment) impact health inequalities?

References

Alderwick, H Hutchings, A and Mays, N (2022) A cure for everything and nothing? Local partnerships for improving health in England. *British Medical Journal*, 378.

Alley, DE Asomugha, CN, Conway, PH and Sanghavi, DM (2016) Accountable health communities—addressing social needs through Medicare and Medicaid. *New England Journal of Medicine*, 374(1): 8–11.

Alston, P (2018) *Statement on Visit to the United Kingdom, by Professor Philip Alston, United Nations Special Rapporteur on Extreme Poverty and Human Rights*. London, UK: United Nations Human Rights Office of the High Commissioner.

Anderson, M Pitchforth, E Edwards, N Alderwick, H McGuire, A and Mossialos, E (2022) United Kingdom: health system review. *World Health Organisation*, 24(1): 1–194.

Bambra, C (2012) Reducing health inequalities: new data suggest that the English strategy was partially successful. *Journal of Epidemiology Community Health*, 66(7): 662–662.

Barr, B Taylor-Robinson, D and Whitehead, M (2012) Impact on health inequalities of rising prosperity in England 1998–2007, and implications for performance incentives: longitudinal ecological study. *British Medical Journal*: 345.

Bochel, H and Powell, M (eds) (2016) *The Coalition Government and Social Policy: Restructuring the Welfare State.* Available at: https://doi.org/10.1332/policypress/9781447324560.001.0001 (accessed 19 July 2024).

Braveman, P and Egerter, S (2008) *Overcoming Obstacles to Health.* USA: Robert Wood Johnson Foundation.

Braveman, PA Egerter, SA and Mockenhaupt, RE (2011) Broadening the focus: the need to address the social determinants of health. *American Journal of Preventive Medicine*, 40(1): S4–S18.

Bywaters, P Skinner, G Cooper, A Kennedy, E and Malik, A (2023) *The Relationship Between Poverty and Child Abuse and Neglect: New Evidence.* London: Nuffield Foundation. Available at: www.nuffieldfoundation.org/wp-content/uploads/2022/03/Full-report-relationship-between-poverty-child-abuse-and-neglect.pdf (accessed 10 June 2024).

Card, AJ (2017) Moving beyond the WHO definition of health: a new perspective for an ageing world and the emerging era of value-based care. *World Medical & Health Policy*, 9(1): 127–137.

Child Poverty Action Group (2022) *We Are the Trusted Voice On Child Poverty.* Available at https://cpag.org.uk (accessed 18 August 2024).

Cooper, K and Stewart, K (2013) *Does Money Affect Children's Outcomes?* York: Joseph Rowntree Foundation.

Crotty, M (1998) *The Foundations of Social Research.* London: SAGE Publications Ltd.

Dahlgren, G and Whitehead, M (2006) *European Strategies for Tackling Social Inequities in Health: Levelling up Part 2.* Denmark: WHO.

Department of Health and Social Care (DHSC) (2022) *Direct and Indirect Health Impacts of COVID-19 in England: Emerging Omicron Impacts.* Available at: www.gov.uk/government/publications/direct-and-indirect-health-impacts-of-covid-19-in-england-emerging-omicron-impacts/direct-and-indirect-health-impacts-of-covid-19-in-england-emerging-omicron-impacts (accessed 29 June 2024).

Department of Health and Social Care (DHSC) (2024) *Annual Report and Accounts 2023–24.* London: DHSC. Available at: https://assets.publishing.service.gov.uk/media/676150 ef26a2d1ff18253415/dhsc-annual-report-and-accounts-2023-2024-web-accessible.pdf (accessed 4 July 2024).

Dunn, P Fraser, C Williamson, S and Alderwick, H (2022) *Integrated Care Systems: What Do They Look Like.* London: Health Foundation.

Dwyer-Lindgren, L Bertozzi-Villa, A Stubbs, RW Morozoff, C Mackenbach, JP Van Lenthe, FJ Mokdad, AH and Murray, CJ (2017) Inequalities in life expectancy among US counties, 1980 to 2014: temporal trends and key drivers. *JAMA Internal Medicine*, 177(7): 1003–1011.

Equality and Human Rights Commission (EHRC) (2023) *Equality and Human Rights Monitor 2023: Executive Summary.* Available at: www.equalityhumanrights.com/our-work/equality-and-human-rights-monitor/equality-and-human-rights-monitor-2023-executive-summary (accessed 25 July 2024).

Faculty of Public Health (2024) *Health Knowledge Resources, Section 3; Concepts of Health and Wellbeing.* Available at: www.healthknowledge.org.uk/public-health-textbook/medical-sociology-policy-economics/4a-concepts-health illness/section2/activity3#:~:text=The%20 WHO%20definition%20links%20health,health%20as%20a%20positive%20aspiration (accessed 19 June 2024).

Ford, J Sowden, S Olivera, J Bambra, C Gimson, A Aldridge, R and Brayne, C (2021) Transforming health systems to reduce health inequalities. *Future Healthcare Journal*, 8(2): 204–209.

Garland, D (2021) The emergence of the idea of 'the welfare state' in British political discourse. *History of the Human Sciences*, 35(1): 132–157.

Garrett, H Mackay, M Simon, N Piddington, J and Roys, M (2021) *The Cost of Poor Housing in England*. Available at: www.https://files.bregroup.com/research/BRE_Report_the_cost_of_poor_housing_2021.pdf (accessed 18 June 2024).

Gibbs, J and Lehtonen, A (2019) I, Daniel Blake (2016): vulnerability, care and citizenship in austerity politics. *Feminist Review*, 122(1): 49–63.

GOV UK (2024) *Understanding and Addressing the Health Risks of Damp and Mould in the Home*. Available at: www.gov.uk/government/publications/damp-and-mould-understanding-and-addressing-the-health-risks-for-rented-housing-providers/understanding-and-addressing-the-health-risks (accessed 4 July 2024).

Health and Care Act 2022, c7.

Huber, M van Vliet, M Giezenberg, M Winkens, B Heerkens, Y Dagnelie, PC and Knottnerus, JA (2016) Towards a 'patient-centred 'operationalisation of the new dynamic concept of health: a mixed methods study. *British Medical Journal*, 6(1).

Huijts, T Eikemo, TA and Skalická, V (2010) Income-related health inequalities in the Nordic countries: examining the role of education, occupational class, and age. *Social Science & Medicine*, 71(11): 1964–1972.

Iliffe, S and Manthorpe, J (2014) A new settlement for health and social care? *British Medical Journal*, 349: 4818.

Institute for Fiscal Studies (2022) *Race and Ethnicity: IFS Deaton Review of Inequalities*. Available at: https://ifs.org.uk/inequality/wp-content/uploads/2022/11/Race-and-ethnicity-IFS-Deaton-Review-of-Inequalities.pdf (accessed 13 July 2024).

Kapadia, D Zhang, J Salway, S Nazroo, J Booth, A Villarroel-Williams, N and Becares, L (2022) *Rapid Review of Ethnic Inequalities and Inequities in Health and Social Care*. NHS Race and Health Observatory. Available at: www.nhsrho.org/wp-content/uploads/2023/05/RHO-Rapid-Review-Final-Report_-.pdf (accessed 29 June 2024).

King's College London (2020) *The Covid Crisis Has Caused Anger, Arguments and Confrontations*. London: King's College London.

Leonardi, F (2018) The definition of health: towards new perspectives. *International Journal of Health Services*, 48(4): 735–748.

Liaqat, R Waseem, M Siddique, HMA and Majeed, MT (2021) Health outcomes of poverty: evidence from around the globe. *Bulletin of Business and Economics*, 10(3): 43–55

Loach, K (2016) *I, Daniel Blake*. [Film] Directed by Ken Loach. UK: Sixteen Films.

Lussenhop, J (2020) How the coronavirus is hitting the US food supply. *BBC News*, 14 April. Available at: www.bbc.co.uk/news/world-us-canada-52311877 (accessed 3 August 2024).

Lynch, SM (2003) Cohort and life-course patterns in the relationship between education and health: a hierarchical approach. *Demography*, 40(2): 309–331.

Macintyre, S Ellaway, A Hiscock, R Kearns, A Der, G and McKay, L (2003) What features of the home and the area might help to explain observed relationships between housing tenure and health? Evidence from the west of Scotland. *Health & Place*, 9(3): 207–218.

MacLeod, G (2018) Introduction: neoliberal urbanism and the spectre of cohesion. *City*, 22(5–6): 647–653. Available at: www.tandfonline.com/doi/full/10.1080/13604813.2018.1507099 (accessed 29 June 2024).

Martino, L (2022) *Concepts of Health, Well-being and Illness, and the Aetiology of Illness: Section 3. Concepts of Health and Well-being*. Available at: www.healthknowledge.org.uk/public-health-textbook/medical-sociology-policy-economics/4a-concepts-health-illness/section2/activity3 (accessed 30 July 2024).

McCartney, G Popham, F McMaster, R and Cumbers, A (2019) Defining health and health inequalities. *Public Health*, 172: 22–30.

Mercer, S Henderson, D Huang, H Donaghy, E Stewart, E Guthrie, B and Wang, H (2021) Integration of health and social care: necessary but challenging for all. *British Journal of General Practice*, 71(711): 442–443

Mind UK (2018) *Health and Social Care Rights*. Available at: www.mind.org.uk/media-a/2905/health-and-social-care-rights-2018.pdf (accessed 12 June 2024).

Mirowsky, J (2017) *Education, Social Status, and Health*. Abingdon: Routledge.

Mirza, HS and Warwick, R (2022) *Race and Ethnicity* (No. R230). IFS Report.

Moller, S and Cai, T (2020) Welfare state policies and their effects. In: Janoski, T de Leon, C Misra, J and Martin I (eds) *The New Handbook of Political Sociology*. Cambridge: Cambridge University Press, pp 812–841.

Parliament UK (2010) Fair society, healthy lives: the Marmot Review. *Strategic Review of Health Inequalities in England Post-2010*. Available at: www.parliament.uk/globalassets/documents/fair-society-healthy-lives-full-report.pdf (accessed 23 September 2024).

Pearson-Stuttard, J Caul, S McDonald, S Whamond, E and Newton, JN (2023) Vaccine coverage and disparities among individuals with diabetes in England: A cross-sectional analysis of primary care data. *The Lancet Public Health*. Available at: www.thelancet.com/action/showPdf?pii=S2666-7762%2823%2900221-1 (accessed 25 July 2024).

Raghupathi, V and Raghupathi, W (2020) The influence of education on health: an empirical assessment of OECD countries for the period 1995–2015. *Archives of Public Health*, 78: 1–18.

Raleigh, V (2023) *The Health of People from Ethnic Minority Groups in England*. The King's Fund. Available at: www.kingsfund.org.uk/insight-and-analysis/long-reads/health-people-ethnic-minority-groups-england (accessed 29 June 2024).

Ro, A Geronimus, A Bound, J Griffith, D and Gee, G (2016) Educational gradients in five Asian immigrant populations: do country of origin, duration and generational status moderate the education-health relationship? *Preventive Medicine Reports*, 4: 338–343.

Royal College of Speech and Language Therapists (2022) *Sustained Impact of COVID-19 Report*. Available at: www.rcslt.org/wp-content/uploads/2022/01/Sustained-Impact-of-COVID-19-Report-RCSLT-January-2022.pdf (accessed 25 July 2024).

Sen, A An, S and Peter, F (2004) Why health equity? In: Anand S, Peter F, and Sen A (eds) *Public Health, Ethics, and Equity*. Oxford: Oxford University Press, pp 21–34.

Schramme, T (2023) Health as complete Well-being: the WHO definition and beyond. *Public Health Ethics*, 16(3): 210–218.

Shilton, T Sparks, M McQueen, D Lamarre, MC and Jackson, S (2011) Proposal for a new definition of health. *British Medical Journal*: 343.

Social Care Institute of Excellence (2014) *What Is an Assessment Under the Care Act?* Available at: www.scie.org.uk/assessment-and-eligibility/assessment-of-needs-under-the-care-act-2014 (accessed 4 Jul 2024).

Sosenko, F Bramley, G and Bhattacharjee, A (2022) Understanding the post-2010 increase in food bank use in England: new quasi-experimental analysis of the role of welfare policy. *Public Health*, 22: 1363.

Taylor-Gooby, P Leruth, B and Chung, H (2017) *After Austerity: Welfare State Transformation in Europe after the Great Recession*. Oxford: Oxford Academic

The King's Fund (2022) *The Health and Social Care White Paper Explained*. Available at. www.kingsfund.org.uk/insight-and-analysis/long-reads/health-social-care-white-paper-explained (accessed 17 August 2024).

The King's Fund (2024) *Social Care in a Nutshell*. Available at: www.kingsfund.org.uk/insight-and-analysis/data-and-charts/social-care-nutshell (accessed 14 June 2014).

Thomas, B Dorling, D and Smith, GD (2010) Inequalities in premature mortality in Britain: observational study from 1921 to 2007. *British Medical Journal*, 341.

Thorlby, R and Maybin, J (2010) *A High-Performing NHS? A Review of Progress 1997–2010*. London: The King's Fund.

Titmuss R (2018) The social division of welfare. In Titmuss, R, *Essays on the Welfare State*. Bristol: Bristol University Press.

Tomaney, J and Pike, A (2020) Levelling up? *The Political Quarterly*, 91(1): 43–48.

Tomas, P and Lynch, P (2023) The black hole in town hall budgets rises to £5bn. *BBC*. Available at: www.bbc.co.uk/news/uk-66428191 (accessed 3 May 2024).

United Nations General Assembly (1948) *Universal Declaration of Human Rights*. Available at: www.un.org/en/universal-declaration-human-rights/ (accessed 3 May 2024).

Wang, Z Wang, J Chen, Z Lu, C Ni, M and Meng, Y (2018) Trends in smoking prevalence and implication for chronic diseases in China: serial national cross-sectional surveys from 2003 to 2013. *British Medical Journal*, 8(10).

Whitehead, M (1992) The concepts and principles of equity and health. *International Journal of Health Services*, 22(3): 429–445.

WHO (World Health Organization) (2025) *Constitution*. Available at: https://www.who.int/about/governance/constitution (accessed 3 April 2025).

World Population Review (2021) *High Income Countries*. Available at: https://world-populationreview.com/country-rankings/high-income-countries (accessed 30 June 2024).

Zajacova, A and Lawrence, EM (2018) The relationship between education and health: reducing disparities through a contextual approach. *Annual Review of Public Health*, 39: 273–289.

Zimmerman, E and Woolf, SH (2014) *Understanding the Relationship Between Education and Health*. Washington: National Academy of Sciences.

Index

Page numbers in *italics* indicate a figure, **bold** a table

For Product Safety Concerns and Information please contact our EU
representative GPSR@taylorandfrancis.com
Taylor & Francis Verlag GmbH, Kaufingerstraße 24, 80331 München, Germany